The Healing Power
of Movement

Also by Lisa Hoffman

Better Than Ever: The Four-Week Workout Program for Women Over 40

The Healing Power of Movement

How to Benefit from Physical Activity During Your Cancer Treatment

Lisa Hoffman, M.A.,
with Alison Freeland

PERSEUS PUBLISHING

Cambridge, Massachusetts

Copyright © 2002 by Lisa Hoffman and Alison Freeland

Cataloging-in-Publication Data is available from the Library of Congress
ISBN 0–7382–0540–0

Perseus Publishing is a member of the Perseus Books Group.
Visit us on the World Wide Web at http://www.perseuspublishing.com.
Perseus Publishing books are available at special discounts for bulk purchases in the United States by corporations, institutions, and other organizations. For more information, please contact the Special Markets Department at the Perseus Books Group, 11 Cambridge Center, Cambridge, MA 02142, or call (800) 255-1514 or (617) 252–5298, or e-mail j.mccrary@perseusbooks.com.

Text design by Reggie Thompson
Illustrations by Meryl Henderson
Set in 11-point Berling Roman by Perseus Publishing Services

First printing, January 2002

1 2 3 4 5 6 7 8 9 10—04 03 02

In memory of those
who have included movement
to heal and gave dignity to their battle.

Vitality shows not only the ability to persist
but the ability to start over.
—F. Scott Fitzgerald

A Note To The Reader

The ideas, exercises, and suggestions contained in this book are not intended as a substitute for consulting with your physician or as medical advice. All matters regarding your health require medical supervision. All readers should consult with a physician before proceeding with these exercises or suggestions. Any undertaking of the exercises or suggestions in this book is at the reader's discretion and sole risk.

Contents

Foreword

Decades ago, rehabilitation and quality of life were not the integral aspects of cancer care that they are today. We were unable to focus on living well with and after cancer because too few patients survived the diagnosis. Today we have that luxury. Close to 60 percent of Americans with cancer are cured. Literally millions of people in the United States right now are under cancer treatment, in rehabilitation, or working to prevent recurrence of their disease.

This book is about improving their strength and enhancing their quality of life. It is a guide for those who have been diagnosed with cancer, who receive or have completed treatment, and who are working their way back to normal, active lives. It offers encouragement and guidance, showing patients that a level of beneficial exercise can be accomplished no matter where they are in the battle against this difficult complex of diseases.

Lisa Hoffman has developed creative exercises for every person facing cancer. Described in words as well as easy-to-follow illustrations, her book is based on substantial experience and shows great sensitivity to the difficulties, motivation, and restrictions experienced by cancer patients. These exercise regimens can be accomplished at every level, from diagnosis through treatment and recovery.

This book is also a testament to the fact that patients have active, important roles to play in their own recovery. Exercise is an important component. Exercising to rebuild strength, flexibility, and coordination provides us with a powerful means of control. We can contribute importantly to our own recovery. Exercise also releases endorphins and makes us feel better—it enhances quality of life in several dimensions.

A professional treatment regimen should be part of every patient's recovery program. The value of this book lies in its careful, creative presentation of a program that can fit the needs and capabilities of every cancer patient, regardless of stage of treatment or rehabilitation. It is a great way to begin and an excellent guide all along the road to recovery.

—*Barrie R. Cassileth, Ph.D.*
Chief, Integrative Medicine Program
Memorial Sloan-Kettering Cancer Center, New York

A Note from Dr. Stephen Nimer

Recently at the hospital we held what we call a survivors' party for patients who have undergone cancer treatment with us. Five hundred people attended, and what a joyful occasion it was. Instead of focusing on their illness, they were focusing on getting back to normal living. For many of them, the issues of how they are dealing with their self-image, their sex drive, and their family relationships are paramount. For many, the topic of the evening was the role of exercise in their life.

There's no question that the medical world's attitude toward illness and exercise has changed in the last decade. For one thing, recuperation time after most surgeries has shortened. Our procedures have improved, and with that, the time it takes for someone to get out of bed and moving has shortened as well.

Additionally, the prevailing mindset used to be "stay in bed and rest as long as possible." Now it's "get up and get around, and it will actually speed your recovery." We encourage patients to get up and move around, even if it's just a walk down the hall, for many reasons. Moving around helps prevent pneumonia that can come with too much bed rest. It helps digestion and stimulates a few endorphins that give a sense of well-being. I can't state unequivocally that activity improves the immune system, but I know it helps fight depression and the feeling that you've lost all control over your life.

When I recommend activity for someone in cancer therapy, I'm not talking about pushing as hard as Lance Armstrong did. Athletes push beyond their endurance as a matter of course. I'm talking about helping yourself maintain a level of fitness. I'm not even looking for you to improve your fitness level, just to maintain it.

Now and then a cancer patient may fear that by being active, they may cause the cancer to actually spread through the body. There is no truth to that fear whatsoever, and pushing the body, not to the point of pain, but to the point of tiredness, is completely safe.

Of course, there are conditions that could preclude you from exercising. If your blood count or platelets are very low, there could be severe bleeding if you were to fall. If your bone density were seriously compromised by illness, you wouldn't want to risk fracturing a bone. However, if bone disease is not an issue, improving your muscle tone will actually increase your chances of not hurting your bones. I wouldn't always recommend weight lifting, but lifting your own body weight is helpful.

Overall, my goal for patients is to see them resume a normal life. For many of them it means being able to play tennis, ski, or run five miles. For many others it means having the strength to run for a bus, climb to the second floor of the house, or pick up a grandchild. There is no reason not to start some kind of activity as soon as you can during and after cancer treatment, and the exercises in this book are a marvelous way to begin.

—*Dr. Stephen Nimer*
Head, Division of Hematologic Oncology
Chief, Hematology Services
Memorial Sloan-Kettering Cancer Center, New York

Preface

Since 1990, I have trained hundreds of men and women with varied health conditions, fitness goals, and motivations. But nothing in my training prepared me for the physical and emotional complexity of working with people fighting for their lives because of cancer.

Special health conditions weren't foreign to me. For over a decade I have trained people to cope with and modify activities for certain health situations. Mostly the modifications were for osteoporosis, rheumatoid arthritis, hip replacements, or even tennis elbow. Cancer, however, brought a whole new meaning to the term "training."

As an exercise physiologist and modern dancer, I have always been interested in how movement can fulfill and enhance physical health, mental well-being, body awareness, and even creative expression. Basically, I worked with people who had a similar interest—people who can't imagine even two days going by without setting off some endorphins while they exercised. They may take classes in a gym, walk, run, or practice tai chi.

When working with people who have cancer, however, I've also discovered others who have no history of wanting to exercise. As a so-called motivator of movement, how do I begin to teach and encourage people with a diagnosis of cancer to regularly participate in physical activity during this time no matter which category they fit in? And so the challenge begins not only for the clients, but for their physicians too. It may be new for the oncologists as well to encourage their patients to be as active as possible during treatment. It may not seem so foreign for avid exercisers to continue to move through their treatment, but for those who have never been interested, how, in fact, can it start now?

What is the appropriate exercise program during treatment, especially when fatigue and nausea can be overwhelming side effects? The program itself has to match one's current energy level, mood, strength, and skill. While I was researching for this book, I came across over forty-three studies that had substantiated the fact that physical activity during cancer treatment is beneficial to one's overall physical function and well-being. This opinion comes from evidence-based research.

This brings me to my next point. Medication is discovered and proven through research. Exercise programs are tried out and proven or disproved as a viable quality-of-life intervention through clinical studies. This is how we benefit and plan our medication treatment protocol or exercise program. Advances in medicine and science are results of new ideas and approaches developed through research. New cancer treatments must prove to be safe and effective in scientific studies with a certain number of patients before they can be made widely available. Then they must withstand critical review by other scientists (known as peer review) in order to be published results in peer-reviewed medical and scientific journals. They are designed to demonstrate that a particular new surgical procedure, radiation or chemotherapeutic treatment, dietary change, or exercise approach has a significant advantage over customary care.

The gold standard of research is the randomized, double-blind clinical trial. In this trial, people are randomly assigned either to a group receiving the experimental treatment, or to a control group, which receives the conventional treatment, a placebo, or nothing. In the case of a double-blind research study design, neither the participants nor the researcher knows which subjects are in the experimental group and which subjects are in the control group. This is to minimize any bias that may happen on either end. By comparing the effects of treatment on both groups, scientists can determine whether the experimental treatment is better than the conventional treatment.

If you or your family member already has cancer, then enrolling in a study may be of interest. Consider asking your physician if there is a study right for you. Maybe there is an exercise physiologist in your cancer center doing a study on quality of life and activity while you are there. Or your physician may be interested in new treatments that have had positive results in the past and will ask you if you would like to partake in a study. With the emergence of new treatments, screening techniques, and decoding of the human genome, questions are beginning to be answered at a rapid pace. Perhaps a clinical trial is right for you.

Cancer is nothing short of a life-threatening illness with an uncertain prognosis with often devastating treatments. It's a shake-up for the patient and his or her family, friends, and coworkers. From diagnosis forward, a new person has evolved—someone living with cancer. Learning to live now with a certain level of ambiguity and vulnerability is part of your life. Let movement be a means of coping, strengthening, and progressing to the vital person you will be again.

I hope this book helps you get moving even when you're in bed most of the day. I hope it helps you regain strength and function when you're feeling better, and helps to motivate you, knowing that physical activity will make you feel better in the short and long term. And, most of all, I hope it helps you heal.

Introduction

*W*HEN PEOPLE THINK OF PERSONAL TRAINERS, they envision a world of hard bodies and calorie counting, of spandex outfits and mirrors in the gym. Although there is a place for that in our society, the kind of personal training I've been involved with for the last ten years is another world entirely. For many years, I've been an exercise physiologist for a special group of clients whose motivation is not vanity but survival. The clients who make up my business may not be able to do even one push-up, and their victories are measured in inches instead of miles. They are all ages and from all professions, but they have one thing in common—cancer stole a part of their life, and they want it back.

In 1999, Lance Armstrong won a stunning victory in the Tour de France after undergoing surgery and chemotherapy for testicular cancer. After his even more impressive second victory a year later and more to follow, the world at large began to acknowledge what many of us in the health industry have suspected for a long time: Exercise rather than rest may be the best thing for someone undergoing cancer therapy. Soon after Armstrong's first victory, the Associated Press carried the message of new research in the field. According to Colleen Doyle, director of nutrition and physical activity for the American Cancer Society, the new research is promising enough that the society is revising its exercise recommendations.

At the advent of this new approach to cancer therapy, I already have a decade of working with people who have proven that such an approach works. *The Healing*

Power of Movement is based on my experience with people who have made moderate exercise a part of their cancer therapy—the quietly brave souls who sometimes count the walk to the gym the sum total of what they can do that day. Their words and their discoveries have fueled this book.

In addition, because of my interaction with doctors at Memorial Sloan-Kettering Cancer Center in New York City and other hospitals, I've been able to incorporate medical research and precautions into the exercise regimens I design for our clients. Their words are also a part of this book.

Inspirations for This Book

Elaine is a typical client of Solo Fitness, my personal training company based in New York City. I think of Elaine as a New York type, but I know there are Elaines all across the country. In her early fifties, she is a no-nonsense partner in an investment firm and a no-nonsense fitness client as well. She had already worked with another personal trainer when I met her and was consistent, demanding, and well versed concerning her physical training. Her business self spilled over into the gym, and I was impressed by how she would set goals for herself, get clear on how to achieve them, and then get to work.

Sessions with Elaine usually had a no-dilly-dally, let's-get-going tempo. If she worked on her legs and felt the left side didn't get as much work as her right, she'd do it over again. "Let's do more," she'd say to me. "I didn't feel it yet." Elaine was into strenuous workouts, and when I was with her we pushed hard.

By Christmas of our first year working together, Elaine experienced a persistent sore throat, and over the next few months it just seemed to worsen. By spring she was diagnosed with leukemia. I went to see her in the hospital when she started her chemotherapy treatments, and I brought a funny book for her. She was still Elaine, conducting so many business calls from her bed that I eventually had to leave without getting to talk to her.

It was many months before I saw Elaine again, and I have to admit I gasped when she walked into the room. It wasn't just the weight loss or the fact that she was bald that made her so different. It was her movements. This strong, decisive woman had become cautious. Finally I noticed her bright blue eyes and said to myself, "Oh, thank heavens. She's still in there."

Elaine began to describe her limitations to me. She had undergone a stem cell transplant procedure and felt frequent dizziness and nausea. Like many people in cancer therapy, she had mind-numbing fatigue. When she got out of bed, she was afraid of going down stairs because her legs might buckle and she'd lose her balance. Her nails were coming off, so she had to be careful what she grabbed. Sitting down and getting up were difficult, and she couldn't take baths because she couldn't get in and out of the tub. She had been embarrassed by not being able to get out of the backseat of a taxi. Her clothes were double-hung on two levels in her clothes closet and she had trouble reaching the top rack.

"I have to get on a step stool to reach my jackets," she moaned. "And I don't want to lose my balance." I looked in the closet and assured her that if she fell, she'd only land in a pile of clothes. For a moment she almost laughed, and I knew we had begun to work together again.

Before I did anything with Elaine, I spoke with her doctor about what we were planning to do. The word *exercise* seems to scare everyone. I knew the doctor suspected I would get Elaine on a trampoline or make her run a mile, and so I talked about activity instead. "I mean we're going to work on getting out of a chair," I explained. "My goal is for Elaine to be able to pick up a towel if she drops it on the bathroom floor, to turn around if someone calls her name, to hoist her purse on her shoulder. That's my goal."

When I worked with Elaine, I had already learned a great deal about fitness for people who have been debilitated by disease. A major portion of our clientele with Solo Fitness have osteoporosis or a fracture or are at risk of this bone-thinning disease. I was used to fine-tuning a program to suit a person's limitations. I began to focus on lower body strength with Elaine so she could stand up and sit down easily. We worked with low ankle weights, building up the muscles that had atrophied in the hospital. I helped her regain range of motion in her ankle joints and flexibility in her torso. The hardest part for her was her frustration at her own condition. Knowing where she'd been before, she was devastated that she couldn't even lift a small weight.

The way Elaine and I got through those first sessions was by laughing and talking together and by my refusal to focus on what she'd lost. She would bend her arms several times in a row and I'd say, "Look, Elaine, you're moving again." Instead of hating how weak she was, she would just try to do it again. If she couldn't lie on her side because she was sensitive from having bone marrow extracted, we did exercises from her knees or from a sitting position.

A year later much of the old Elaine was back again. Her hair grew in and she regained muscle tone. When she bent her arms to do bicep curls, she again held eight-pound weights, and when she went for a walk in the park, she did it without fear that fatigue would overwhelm her and keep her from making it back home. Recently she stood up and sat down twenty times for me without using her hands for help, and one night she called to tell me she had taken her first bath.

Elaine is one of many individuals who keep teaching me how to work with people recovering from cancer. Another one of our clients has multiple myeloma. She opened the door the first time I met her, and I was struck by how fragile she was, as if she might break either physically or mentally. She reminded me of a tree in the middle of winter, bare of leaves and spindly. We began our first session by standing near the wall and placing our palms flat against the surface. She was tentative about even doing that much. Then we pressed a little bit. A while later I put her on a stationary bicycle. She never pedaled, and I never turned it on. I just held her there.

Many fitness trainers track their clients' progress by the energy exerted, the weight lost, or the obvious improvement in someone's ability to lift weights or work on a treadmill. Working with a client with cancer, I track progress in different increments. Did the client laugh today? That's a big deal. Were they able to carry their own towel and hand weight to the gym? That's progress. Did they feel safe and stable on their feet? That's a great day. Did they leave our time together feeling uplifted? That's victory.

When I work with people who have been through chemotherapy, radiation treatment, stem cell or bone marrow transplants, hormone therapy, and surgery, I throw out all the benchmarks I used to hold for our other clients. When a person is at their weakest, sometimes we just press palms together and call it a day. Today I'm gratified if the person makes it through a session without having to be sick or lean against the wall or cry. I know that any amount of activity is beneficial both physically and mentally and helps contribute to a feeling of control.

We can thank Lance Armstrong for making people conscious of a new way of dealing with cancer therapy and exercise. For years the medical profession felt the human body was working hard enough just fighting cancer. The only activity they recommended was relaxation techniques or gentle stretching.

One of our clients, Matthew, was completely frustrated when his doctor told him not to run anymore when he was diagnosed with cancer. Running was how Matthew relaxed and how he worked out issues. To be forbidden to run when he still felt well was a blow. Matthew inspired my original research into physical activity during cancer treatment. As far as I could find, there was no need to stop all activity when undergoing therapy. After reviewing the literature with me, he made the decision to stay as active as possible and to take each day as it came. Matthew was able to run on the treadmill for the majority of his treatment. Even though his five-mile run turned into a one-mile run and a two-mile walk, he continued to do what made him comfortable and happy.

Then the world watched in 1999 as Lance Armstrong won the Tour de France cycling race and wore the winner's yellow jersey. Three years earlier, Lance had been diagnosed with testicular cancer and had surgery to remove a diseased testicle. His nightmare intensified when they found that the cancer had spread to his vital organs. He went through chemotherapy.

The remarkable aspect to Lance's story is that while coming back from chemotherapy treatments, he began training again. He rode at least fifty miles a day. He was fortunate and trained well enough to race in the Tour de France, and then he won. To come back not just to riding again, but to race in the most demanding competition, and then to win, was visible evidence that not only would exercise not hurt someone recovering from cancer—it might help them regain their normal life.

Lance Armstrong became a vivid example of what health professionals had already started to realize—keeping active during and after cancer treatment at worst causes no harm, and at best can improve quality of life and perhaps speed recovery. Obviously, there are considerations depending on a person's age, type of illness, and factors such as blood counts and level of physical fitness to begin with. Few people would think of cycling fifty miles a day even when they were totally healthy. Nevertheless, there is an emerging sense that maintaining some kind of activity during and after cancer treatment is important. The question is, how to go about it?

The how of staying active through your treatment is where this book comes in. The activity suggestions and philosophy in this book come from my experience as an exercise physiologist. The information is a combination of what was learned from my own research, our clients' experiences, and doctors' suggestions.

It's now been over ten years since the first time I worked with someone who had cancer. This book came about because of all the Elaines and Matthews, and the countless other brave and funny souls I've worked with during this time, who have taught me that sometimes just putting one foot in front of the other is a major victory.

1

How to Use This Book

THE HEALING POWER OF MOVEMENT is a step-by-step guide to help a person undergoing cancer treatment begin to move again and to find a level of activity that helps them energize. I think of it as the book a cancer patient will want to keep close at hand for motivation and direction. The chapters address people who can barely move from their beds, all the way through to those who are walking and jogging and resuming a normal life.

When someone walks out the hospital door after each cancer treatment, he or she also walks away from the medical staff that is there to help and answer questions. The patient goes back to a home and life, often with depleted energy, frightening side effects from drugs, and specific limitations to movement. *The Healing Power of Movement* is like having a personal trainer in the house with suggestions on how to approach a reasonable exercise regimen, someone who can relate to the incremental steps of progress common to those being treated for cancer.

This book includes specific exercises for different stages of cancer treatments and for different types of cancers, clearly illustrated. The book includes input from cancer specialists as well as input from the fitness trainers in my company who have been working with cancer patients to formulate personal routines and ways around their unique limitations.

Not everyone can hire a personal trainer to come in and work with them during an illness. Therefore, I've included in this book activities for you to do on your own and with a partner. There are suggestions for the bedridden and for those who can move about the room. I've marked activities for special conditions such as dizziness or when one part of the body is specifically affected by surgery. In each section I've included warnings about conditions that might make the activity dangerous.

The Healing Power of Movement includes the voices of many of the people who have helped me develop these programs. The cancer specialists at Memorial Sloan-Kettering Cancer Center in New York City have contributed their understanding of what is appropriate activity for cancer patients. The Solo Fitness trainers contributed their collective knowledge of what it is to work with people whose physical bodies have been impaired.

All readers will want to review the chapters "Exercise and Cancer Therapy" and "How Much Should I Exercise?" Then, depending on the stage of your cancer therapy, choose the chapter of activities that best reflects how much you're able to move.

Recently I became involved with an organization in New York City called Miracle House. As in many other areas near large hospitals, Miracle House offers out-of-town patients who have an extended treatment at the hospital a place to live. When I first made my services available at Miracle House, I met a man named Jimmy who came from Florida to have specialized cancer therapy in New York. Jimmy was used to working outdoors, and the closeness of Manhattan's buildings coupled with the fatigue from the drugs he was taking was giving him the added problem of depression.

Again, it was one of my clients who taught me some important lessons. When I began working with Jimmy, his wife sat to one side watching. This was a couple who had been together for many years, and having her as an observer seemed distant and awkward to all of us. Soon Jimmy's wife was involved with our activity, and I learned about the importance of inviting a partner to help with these exercises. It was also with Jimmy that I added music to the regimen. After a session involving all three of us moving to music in a small New York bedroom, Jimmy was able to laugh and admit that he felt more like himself.

I encourage you to follow our example. If there is a partner or caretaker in your life who can help you follow an exercise routine, it will make it all the easier to accomplish. And music is an essential ingredient. Choose the most upbeat music you can find, and see if it doesn't help lift you from the bed.

2

Exercise and Cancer Therapy

CLINICAL STUDIES FROM THE LAST DECADE are starting to show what I've seen on a small scale for a long time: *moderate physical activity is a progressive new method for rehabilitating cancer patients.* It has been shown in numerous studies that structured physical activity helps a cancer patient be able to do activities of daily living with less effort, to cope with fatigue, to increase aerobic capacity, and to counter the effects of inactivity and help fight depression, still feeling in control of one's body. As more cancer practitioners encourage their patients to become active, the benefits are becoming clearer.

More and more people are cancer survivors owing to early detection, more effective screening, and improved quality of treatment. Whatever can contribute to quality of life for you during treatment and recovery is essential. People are looking for ways to combat the side effects of treatment and help maintain some sort of normalcy during this very erratic and intrusive time of life. Both researchers and physicians are looking into the importance of staying active and functional through cancer treatment.

Moderate physical activity such as walking on a treadmill, cycling (continuous or intermittent), light weights, relaxation techniques, and stretching can all help maintain physical function, combat fatigue, and decrease nausea and neuropathy in the short term. In the long term, it can diminish consequences of cancer treatment such as early menopause because of cancer therapy or the increased risk of osteoporosis.

Maybe most important, light exercise enables one to be proactive during cancer treatment.

As suggested by prominent sports medicine researcher Dr. Fernando Dimeo, being physical during this difficult, scary, and unnerving time may not be possible throughout your recovery. For instance, you need to watch for times when your platelet count is too low or you are just too nauseous from your medication or if it is too difficult to eat and drink sufficiently to maintain energy. The overall aim is not to give you a hard body or to help you train for a marathon, but simply to get you up and functioning during your therapy rather than delaying movement until your therapy is completed.

You may have heard of possible dangers to physical exercise during cancer treatment, or you may have thought up some all on your own. Until recently, doctors looked at the fatigue experienced by many cancer patients and told them to rest as much as possible, trying to help them conserve precious energy for only the most necessary activities. Research data indicates, however, that the absence of activity may generate its own effects of impairment and that the only way to begin overcoming fatigue is to start moving.

A fear some patients have is that physical exertion will somehow cause their cancer to spread around the body, a worry that doctors say is medically groundless. A concern doctors have had, however, is that physical activity might depress the body's natural killer cells (NKCs) and thus damage the body's natural cancer-fighting defenses. NKCs are important in combating viral infections and cancer. Data suggest that both cancer history and stress may be associated with reductions in NKC activity. However, continuous long-term moderate exercise has been shown to enhance the immune system; only extreme exercise can have an ill effect on the NKCs.

We all know that many people with cancer have as hard a fight with the disease mentally as they do physically. The shock of hearing the diagnosis, combined with fear and the foreignness of the hospital environment, makes for a real life-changer for anyone in the situation. It's almost certain you'll experience depression over both the illness and the treatment as well as some sense of losing control over your life. Add to that the bone-deep fatigue and possible loss of movement because of surgery, and you may feel that you barely know yourself anymore.

Nevertheless, even moderate activity can begin to reverse the most debilitating mental effects of the disease. First of all, being able to perform a routine exercise gives you one place in your life where you begin to regain control. Instead of being a passive recipient of all kinds of drug and surgical therapies, you can begin to be an active participant in your recovery. Second, and ironically, moderate activity tends to give you energy instead of depleting it. After exercising, you will feel more like getting up and doing something than if you had lain in bed for the same amount of time. Additionally, exercise fights off the bad effects of inactivity such as muscle weakness, loss of energy, and stiffness. Last, one effect of exercise seems to be an increased ability to control your moods. This is where the hard-to-define term "quality of life" comes in. If exercise helps reduce anxiety even a little bit, it becomes an essential component of your life every day.

Recent medical studies have taken patients with different types of cancer and had some of them do moderate exercising during their treatment. In most cases the exercise consisted of aerobic activity such as stationary bicycling or walking on a treadmill, increased over time. The control group didn't exercise. In each case[1] (the studies are listed below), the people who exercised showed better results than the control group, especially in the quality-of-life arena. Even moderate exercise helped people function at a higher level in their daily life. This could mean anything from an increased ability to make it up the stairs after a meal to being able to carry out simple chores like bringing in the mail or taking the dog for a walk.

Exercise enhances recovery and doesn't hinder the immune system or other bodily systems such as cardiac or respiratory functions. The results of the clinical studies, in brief, show that exercise is not dangerous, but in fact improves your overall health and well-being.

In this book, I want to help you find the motivation and the method to begin some kind of physical activity during your cancer treatment. The critical issue is to figure out the optimal level of activity that you can perform with the lowest risk. Exercise guidelines are given for specific cancers and their considerations.

---

[1]Studies cited for exercise during cancer treatment: MacVicar, 1989; Dimeo, 1996; Mock, 1994; Brennan, 1998; Pedersen, 1995; Nieman, 1995.

For example, if a side effect of your surgery is lymphedema in one of your arms, there are ways to address that problem and concentrate on the other arm. Perhaps you are dealing with bone cancer and have pain associated with weight-bearing activities; then I suggest other ways to exercise that you can do while lying down or sitting in a chair. Individual programs are explained to make the most out of your physical activity. There is no medical reason to wait until after your treatment to start moving again. Starting sooner rather than later will offset the bad effects of inactivity, help you regain confidence and control, and most likely help elevate your mood and your outlook on life. With that as the goal, there's no time like the present to start.

3

How Much Should I Exercise?

*T*HERE IS NOT ONE ULTIMATE EXERCISE prescription for cancer patients at various stages of the disease. Right now there are not even explicit standards for the type, frequency, duration, intensity, or progression of exercise for people in cancer treatment. However, we can make confident recommendations drawn from the growing body of research studies of the last ten years. Above all, studies conclude that exercise is safe, feasible, and beneficial to anyone's quality of life at almost any stage of cancer therapy. Of course, there are considerations if you have a severe physical impairment, a condition such as anemia, or a particular part of your body that is limited because of surgery, but they are just that—considerations—not reasons to avoid activity.

Although the focus of *The Healing Power of Movement* is to promote physical activity, there may be mitigating factors that make exercise unwise or dangerous for a few individuals. Some patients may benefit from a supervised exercise program, and close medical supervision may be required for others.

There may be times during your treatment that you don't feel like exercising. These down days are different for each person and may vary from cycle to cycle. The key is to listen to your body and modify the frequency, intensity, or duration of any exercise. As you go through treatment, you will get used to hearing a lot of numbers associated with your condition. You will have your blood counts and heart function checked regularly in addition to receiving nutritional guidance. As for the

Contraindications and Restrictions to Exercise

Red blood cells ≤ 10 mg/Hb (normal count is 12–14 mg/Hb)
Platelets ≤ 50,000 cells per microliter
Neutrophils ≤ 1,000 cells per microliter
White blood cells ≤ 3,000 cells per microliter (normal count is in 5,000–10,000 range)
Fever > 100° F
Muscle weakness
Numbness in the extremities
Extreme fatigue
Pain
Nausea
Dizziness
Dehydration
Day of surgery/treatment

numbers above, they should be used only as a guideline and should not be substituted for a physician's supervision.

The American College of Sports Medicine (ACSM) has set guidelines for the general population, and people in cancer treatment may closely follow the same suggestions. The guidelines call for exercising three to five days a week, twenty to thirty minutes per session.

What Kind of Exercise?

Mountain climbing, running, playing tennis? The most important point is that the exercise feels right to you. You have to use your instinct as to which activities you want to perform. While you're in cancer therapy you probably won't take up a sport you've never attempted before, and any activity you attempt has to be modified for the treatment effects of surgery, chemotherapy, or radiation.

Let me start by saying that walking and cycling are the two activities recommended most often because they are safe and tolerable for the majority of people. Doctors who have studied cancer treatment and exercise have concentrated on exercises for the large muscle groups, and concentrated on exercises that are easily measured. Walking is a natural choice because it relates to all of the activities of daily living that anyone recovering from a disease looks forward to doing.

Most of the medical studies concerning cycling were done in a hospital setting, and cycling proves to be a good choice for most recovering patients. Some studies were even done while the patients were bedridden and only able to move their legs. Swimming has proven to be another safe aerobic activity that promotes cardiovascular and overall fitness. However, if your cancer therapy includes catheters or nephrostomy tubes, swimming may not be appropriate for you. Good sense would tell you that if you are recovering from primary or metastatic bone cancer, high-impact or contact sports are out of the question.

Can I Exercise Too Much?

There is some evidence that repeated, high-intensity exercise could lower your immune system and therefore be unsafe if you are recovering from surgery or chemotherapy. Dr. Fernando Dimeo suggests you will want to keep your heart rate under 75 percent of maximum (subtract your age from 220 to get your maximum heart rate). On the other hand, unless you have been a professional athlete, it is unlikely that you will want to push yourself to this extreme during cancer treatment. Once you've rebounded from treatment, however, and returned to your normal workload and lifestyle, there is no evidence that high-intensity exercise isn't appropriate.

Can I Vary the Exercises?

Many researchers in this field recommend intermittent or interval training. This means short bouts of exercise coupled with rest. If you are in the first stages of recovery from chemotherapy or bone marrow transplants, this intermittent exercise throughout the day is a good way to accumulate your thirty minutes.

As for weight training, studies on the efficacy of this type of exercise are only beginning to come to light. It is likely that the optimal exercise regime for most cancer patients will combine aerobic activity and weight training. The exercises I've recommended in this book offer that combination.

The key to *The Healing Power of Movement* is not just to focus on walking or cycling, but to add specific muscle conditioning to help you maintain the optimal level of function at any given time during your treatment. From my years of experience working with all different kinds of patients and survivors, I've seen that walking alone simply doesn't cut it. Just as for healthy adults who aren't fighting cancer, you will need to combine aerobic activity with muscle conditioning and strengthening, and add stretching as well.

The clinical studies suggest that the sooner you begin to exercise, no matter how feeble the attempt, the sooner you will regain your normal level of functioning. If you allow yourself only rest, you will contribute to further decline of your agility, your energy level, and ultimately to your quality of life. Your question really isn't "can I exercise too much?" but "how can I exercise enough?"

4

From Your Diagnosis Forward

SEVERAL YEARS AGO, ONE OF MY CLIENTS, Gini, was getting ready for a much-needed break at the beach during the last weeks of August. I had worked with Gini twice weekly for three years, mostly doing weight training for specific parts of her body and helping her build endurance on a stationary bike. Gini was in her early fifties and had recovered from surgery for breast cancer that occurred before I knew her. A lawyer by profession, she spent most of her day sitting in a chair. For her, getting up and doing some exercise during the day was welcomed. Standing face-to-face with me, she had a good eight inches on my five-foot-one body. She was always a dynamic presence, authoritative, domineering, and what I call a very styling woman. With short spiky brown hair and clothes that seemed to fall perfectly over her body, she tastefully camouflaged her not-so-perfect waist and arms. Always, Gini was polished and meticulous down to her socks and shoes.

I knew that Gini had undergone a lumpectomy and had a few lymph nodes removed. She had a tendency for lymphedema when she would carry luggage or a heavy package. She was also on medication for both high blood pressure and high cholesterol. At the time of our meeting, she was premenopausal and not thinking of taking hormone replacement therapy for various reasons. This also prompted her to be consistent in her exercise routine to help decrease her risk of heart disease, osteoporosis, and to help her maintain a proper weight, but mostly just to feel good.

That summer, I arrived for our usual workout on a Monday. As far as I knew, Gini and I were winding down before the summer break and putting together a program for her to follow at the beach. I walked into her living room and sat down to check her blood pressure as I always did. She looked at me hesitantly and said, "Lisa, I have cancer again."

As her exercise physiologist, I thought, "What do I say? How do I react? What is the professional response to this?" In the end I only managed to say one word: "Oh," as I realized that from that moment on, our workout schedule, our goals, and our routines would change dramatically.

It takes time to figure out a strategy for fighting cancer, and days go by as you try to cope, cry a little, investigate your options, research, talk, and plan for life with unknown limitations. My job was to provide Gini with a variety of exercises, movements, and stretches that she could handle at the time of each session. For a few weeks, the only perceptible change we dealt with was the diagnosis. Gini didn't feel sick or tired; she couldn't feel cancer. She did, however, feel anxious and confused, and she knew she was facing an ordeal that could take over her life for more than the next few months. My goal became to help her maintain her physicality throughout her treatment.

I continued Gini's basic routine, but I added some walks outside in the park where we would stop to watch schoolchildren play and dogs chase each other in the sunshine. Not only was it enjoyable to get outside during the summer, but walking is also a weight-bearing activity that helps to maintain bone health. We also used these walks as a time to talk about what was to come and to plan for the physical challenges ahead.

Gini's strategy for her breast cancer this time was a mastectomy, and for her breast reconstruction, a TRAM-flap at the same time as her mastectomy. A TRAM-flap procedure stands for transverse rectus abdominus myocutaneous flap. Basically the surgeon takes an area of skin around and below the belly button and transfers it to the place where the breast has been removed. Most commonly the skin and fat remains attached to one or both of the rectus abdominus muscles that provide a blood supply. The abdomen is closed, leaving a scar from hip to hip. The missing muscle is often replaced with a surgical mesh material to reduce the risk of a hernia or bulging of the abdomen. Another part of Gini's treatment strategy would be a regimen of the drug Tamoxifen for five years and having a nipple reconstruction one year after surgery.

In the few weeks between her diagnosis and surgery I added more light stretches to Gini's routine and moments of relaxation at the end of each session. We continued working on her upper body strength because we knew she would have to rely on her arms and legs to get out of bed instead of her abdominal muscles. We also focused on lower back exercises and posture alignment, since after surgery it would probably be difficult to stand upright and walk straight for the first few weeks, which in turn might aggravate her back. We continued her program with stationary bicycling and full-body strength training and stretching. Gini was still able to do just about everything, from bicep curls with five-pound weights to sit-ups and outer thigh lifts. Since she had a history of lymphedema, we did not do any heavy lifting with the affected arm (blood pressure was always taken on the nonaffected arm). We continued to do some upper back work with exercise bands in a sitting position to maintain upper body strength and posture. We began playing classical music in the background while we worked out. Exercising to the sounds of Mozart or Beethoven gave us both an hour of freedom of movement when cancer was a distant thought.

I didn't see Gini again until four weeks after her surgery. She walked tentatively to greet me, and I noticed she was wearing a loose dress that hung over her midsection so it wouldn't irritate her scar. Underneath, she told me, she was wrapped with bandages and her skin was black and blue. Her range of motion around the affected arm was limited, and she talked about being sore all over. She was also having sleepless nights due to night sweats from her Tamoxifen, and because of the incision in her abdominal area, it was hard to get into a comfortable position to sleep. Needless to say, during the first few weeks when we began working together again, she was feeling pretty fatigued and sore. I had already spoken with her doctor and nurses, and after a big hello and a gentle hug, we started a plan of helping Gini stay active through her treatment.

Since part of her abdominal muscle was no longer there but was replaced by strong mesh during her reconstruction surgery, there was a loss of strength and sensation around her midsection. Most movements that one wouldn't think twice about, such as standing up, getting out of bed, or putting on a shirt, became tedious and painful chores. Our exercises focused on everyday life activities, and I sensed that Gini was already becoming an active participant in her own recovery. We began with exercises to restore her shoulder function, then moved on to resolving the back pain that sneaked in at times from her strained posture.

As time went on, the exercise routine gradually changed. From doing light stretches in her chair to prevent scar tissue and maintain an upright position, Gini improved to doing standing exercises, using the wall for support. I could see her strength and confidence return. I began to focus on improving the range of motion of her shoulder joint with exercises we call wall climbs. I learned to help her keep her arm elevated when appropriate and pump her hand to facilitate fluid drainage because of her sensitivity for lymphedema. She continued to strengthen her torso and abdominal area and to do basic leg exercises to support her lower body, as shown in the exercise sections of this book. I made sure Gini stayed away from any heavy lifting for her upper body and any activity that caused pain in her abdominal area. She even included some light exercises while lying in bed, since this was easier for her than lying on the floor.

A few months after surgery, Gini could lie down on a mat and do a series of pelvic tilts and bridges. Her body needed to compensate for the weakness in her abdominal area when transitioning from standing to sitting to lying on the floor and back up again. So it took a bit longer to get down on the floor, using her arms for stability, but once she made it there, I made sure it was worth it. She was able to lie on her stomach with pillow support to perform some basic back exercises. Six months after surgery she performed twisting, or oblique, exercises, and with a select choice of sit-ups (lifting the upper body off the floor by only a few inches) to slowly bring back some abdominal strength without risking any bulging or a hernia. By this time we were taking walks together again and she was confident she could walk away from home and not find herself too fatigued to get back.

It's now been three years since Gini's surgery, and we're still working together. Even though our program has become routine, I am constantly aware of not asking her to do an activity that would aggravate the sites of her surgeries. She can even do sit-ups, in moderation, without any discomfort. There are times here and there that lymphedema occurs, usually after she has been traveling and carrying her luggage. At that point, we shift our exercise focus to more range of motion and stretching exercises and leave the hand weights for another day. She has even started to take a yoga class. She's not able to perform every posture, but her instructor has shown her variations that work for her. And I can certainly see the difference, especially in her alignment, balance, and strength.

I know whenever Gini is facing another check-up at the oncologist's office or another outpatient procedure, because I see the anxiety building in her expressions and in her eyes. We usually use the few days before a doctor's appointment to do simple stretching and relaxation sessions to help her calm her mind. We have both seen that maintaining her exercise routine, no matter what her physical condition, has given her a sense of calm during emotionally trying times, and more important, a sense of control during chaos.

Everyone reacts differently to the diagnosis of cancer, but Gini's example touches on the issues everyone shares in common. Keeping physical activity a part of your life, no matter how bleak the conditions, gives you a tangible way to participate in your treatment and keeps you fit enough to restart your life with a minimum of discomfort.

5

Bed Exercises: Feeling Lousy

Goal: To prepare your body for movement

THE AIM OF BED EXERCISES IS TO HELP YOU avoid the effects of physical inactivity and to improve your physical functioning during cancer therapy rather than delay it until afterward. There's no reason to wait to move until you are done with your treatment. These activities will prepare your body for being active once you're on your feet, even if you're only preparing to walk to the mailbox or to climb some stairs. These exercises also help maintain lean body mass and weight.

You can perform the following exercises in your bed at home or in the hospital when appropriate. This section is for those of you who feel generally lousy, mostly exhausted, and defeated by even the smallest activity. The thought of getting out of bed even to get a glass of water seems like climbing Mount Everest. Perhaps this is a day or two after your chemotherapy, a few days after surgery, or a week after your stem cell or bone marrow transplant. You have spent the majority of the day resting in bed. You may have the added indignity of side effects such as mouth sores, dry skin, or tingling in the feet. Often nausea or dizziness makes standing up impossible.

I've learned a little about what goes through a person's mind at a time like this. I look at someone in your situation and know that you don't think you have the energy to move. What I do know, however, is that movement will actually give you energy. You might remember that it's possible to lift your arm, but it's hard for you to picture it actually happening. You can recall walking across the room to answer the phone or bending down to pick up a piece of paper that has fallen from the table, yet now those simple actions seem to belong to another world.

When you are in this situation, the first challenge to overcome is a mental challenge. You need to find the motivation to attempt movement. It's likely the motivation will come from someone else, and that's why it helps to have a caregiver or a friend or family member who will stand by your bed and encourage you to give it a try. The movement won't hurt you. Continuing to lie motionless will.

Being sedentary has multiple bad effects on the body. Lying down for several weeks can decrease your muscle mass, insulin sensitivity and bone density. You will tend to retain more fluid, and your lung capacity will diminish. (In turn, these put you at increased risk for other health issues.) Psychologically you begin to feel helpless.

The reason I want to get you moving is that activity, no matter how small, will actually give you energy. You'll see, a few days after you start, you'll be able to do more and more and eventually will go on to the next section of this book. The effects of training will take place. Movement stimulates your blood flow and gets more oxygen into your cells. It facilitates glucose metabolism and can help you feel less stiff and lethargic. Movement will do something for your mind as well. It will give you a bit of hope that better times are to come. Remember, small movements, even getting dressed, will help. As one client wrote to us, "Even if we only press hands together, it will be something." Moving helps more than your muscles and joints, it simply makes you feel better. The following activities are for your darkest hours and may be done with the help of a caregiver or loved one.

Plan Your Physical Activity Program

Your doctors have administered the medical treatment, and now it's your turn to participate in your recovery by administering the movement treatment. First of all, ask your physician if there are limitations to an exercise program for you. In addition, get advice on the kind of nutrition you might need to maintain your energy when adding or reintroducing exercise to your daily routine. Begin when you are ready,

---

You want to build muscle strength and stamina to:
- Increase physical function.
- Maintain balance and movement skills for the mechanics of sitting and standing.
- Counter the physiological effects of inactivity and help fight depression by giving you a sense of control over your body.
- Prepare your body for practical daily activities such as picking up your shoes, reaching for a top shelf, being able to feed yourself, going to the bathroom, or getting up and down stairs.

---

and remember that you can take frequent breaks to gather your strength. You're not trying to win a medal; you're trying to prepare your body for when you can stand up again. When that time comes, you don't want to be defeated because you lost critical muscle mass. You want to be able to walk across the room on strong legs.

Normally, when people exercise they are doing it for health benefits and for vanity's sake. Perhaps they are trying to lose weight or stay fit. When we talk about exercise for a cancer patient, the motivation is entirely different. I want to emphasize that movement for a cancer patient is designed to give you energy and to prepare your body for later activity. Contrary to the mantra of "no pain, no gain," cancer patients should not repeat movements if they have significant pain. Additionally, you may have to adapt exercises to accommodate a part of your body that has undergone surgery. One of our clients holds an eight-pound weight in one hand and a two-pound weight in the other because she had breast surgery on one side.

A Note to Caregivers

Many people who have undergone surgery or drug treatment have a weakened immune system. For this reason, it is important for caregivers to wash their hands thoroughly before working with someone, holding them, or helping them move in bed. In some cases the patient you're caring for may be confused as a result of their drug regimen. In other cases they may fall into a well of depression or fear. The goal of doing these bed exercises is as much psychological as physical. If a person can feel the slightest bit of control over their body or have the sense that they can actually do something for themselves, it will be worth the effort.

Deep Breathing/Pelvic Tilts

Benefits: Abdominal muscles, focuses on diaphragmatic breathing and respiration

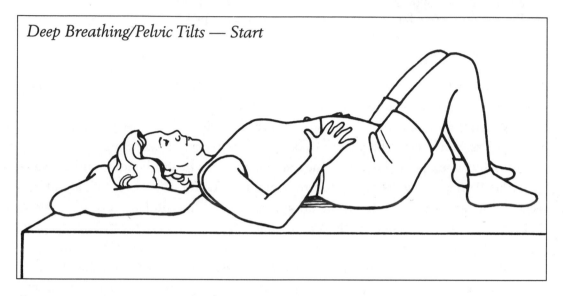

Deep Breathing/Pelvic Tilts — Start

Starting position. Lie on your back with both knees bent, feet flat on the bed, and your hands on your abdomen.

Deep Breathing/Pelvic Tilts — Action

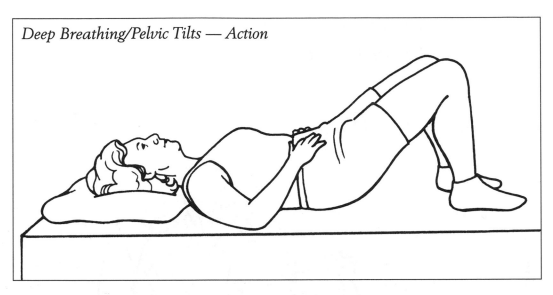

Action.   Inhale and feel your abdominal area rise to the ceiling (feeling a big belly) and exhale while drawing your belly button to the spine, keeping your lower back on the bed.

Notes.   It is beneficial for anyone during cancer treatment, particularly for early postoperative breast surgery patients, to expand your chest cavity, relax and reduce muscle tension in your chest, and enhance lymphatic circulation by moving your diaphragm.

Arm Presses to Ceiling with Partner

Benefits: Pectorals (chest) and arm muscles

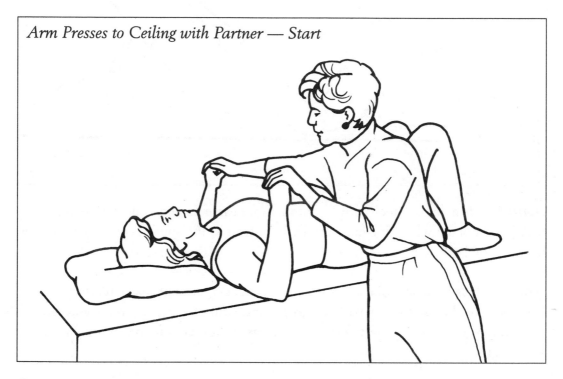

Arm Presses to Ceiling with Partner — Start

Starting position.   Lie on your back with both knees bent and feet flat on the bed. With your arms out to the sides and elbows bent, make a fist with your hands with your palms forward, forearms off the bed. Your partner should be standing next to you with their hands over your fists.

Arm Presses to Ceiling with Partner — Action

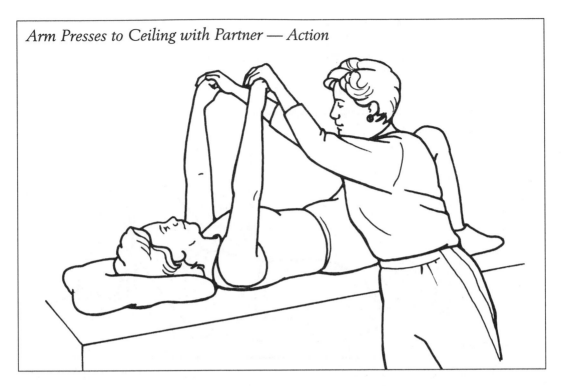

Action. Exhale and extend your arms straight up above your chest, straightening your elbows. Inhale and return to the starting position. Your partner should be giving you slight resistance when you are lifting your hands toward the ceiling. Repeat 5–10 times.

Notes. If your shoulder joint has limited range of motion (ROM) because of surgery or a venous port, please modify the exercise for comfort. This may take some adjusting because of the height of your bed and the height of your partner. Modify as needed. Also, you can elevate your arm to 90 degrees to promote the drainage of lymph fluid. (Avoid raising your arm above shoulder level until about 7 days after surgery with physician approval or when the drains have been removed and it can be done without pain.) Between one and three days following breast surgery, gentle shoulder rotations and lifting the shoulder joints are recommended to promote movement in the shoulder area.

Alternating Knee Lifts

Benefits: Psoas (hip flexor) muscles

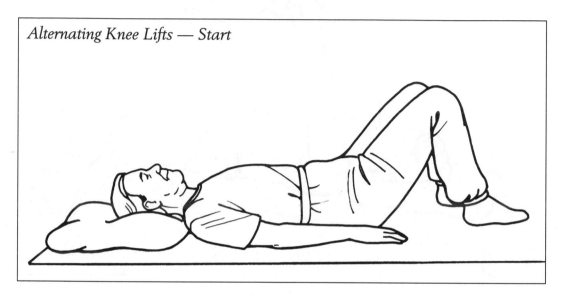

Alternating Knee Lifts — Start

Starting position.   Lie on your back with both knees bent, feet flat on the bed, and your arms at your sides.

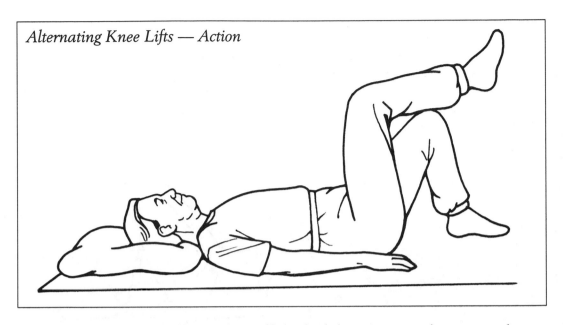

Alternating Knee Lifts — Action

Action. Exhale and lift one foot off the bed, bringing your knee toward your chest. Inhale and return to starting position. Repeat on the other side. Repeat 5–10 times.

Notes. If you have pain in your hip joint because of orthopedic concerns, metastasis, or joint limitation, please modify or refrain from doing this exercise.

Ankle Circles

Benefits: Range of motion in ankle joint, prepare for walking, balance

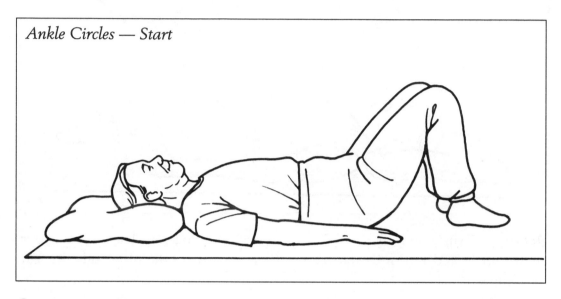

Ankle Circles — Start

Starting position.   Lie on your back with both knees bent, feet flat on the bed, and your arms at your sides.

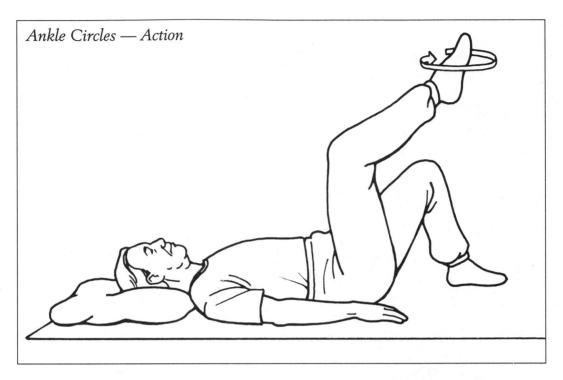

Ankle Circles — Action

Action.   Lift one foot off the bed, bringing your knee toward your chest, and extend your leg slightly toward the ceiling (knee should remain bent). If needed, use your arms to support your leg; circle your ankle. Breathe normally throughout the action. Repeat 5–10 times in each direction with each leg.

Notes.   You may keep your knee bent and your foot low if it is more comfortable for you.

Towel Push-Outs

Benefits: Rhomboid (mid-back), latissimus dorsi (back) muscles

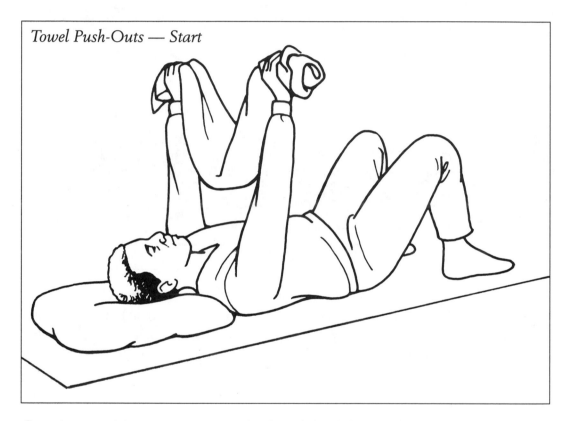

Towel Push-Outs — Start

Starting position.   Lie on your back with both knees bent and your feet flat on the bed. Hold onto a rolled towel by the ends with your hands up to the ceiling.

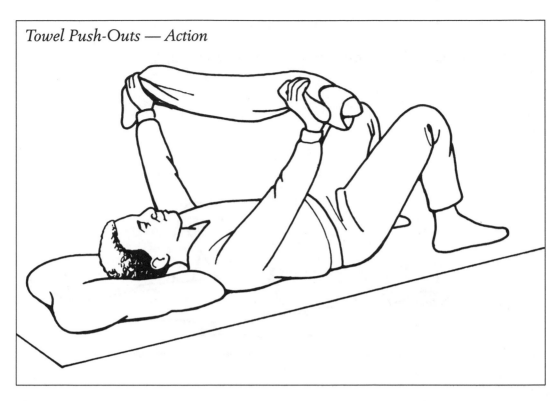

Towel Push-Outs — Action

Action.   Exhale as you extend your arms out to the side, keeping your towel taut, and hold this position for five counts. Inhale and return your arms to the starting position. Repeat 5–10 times.

Notes.   Modify as needed.

Leg Lifts

Benefits: Quadricep (front of thigh) and psoas (hip flexor) muscles

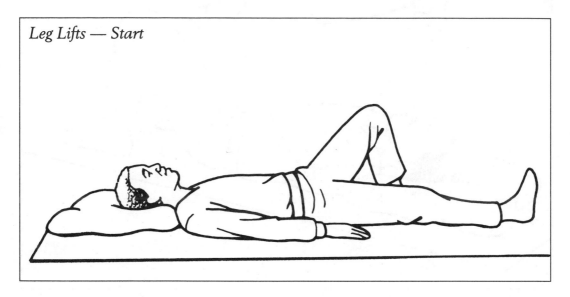

Leg Lifts — Start

Starting position.   Lie on your back with both knees bent, feet flat on the bed, with your arms at your sides. Slide one leg straight down and flex your foot.

Leg Lifts — Action

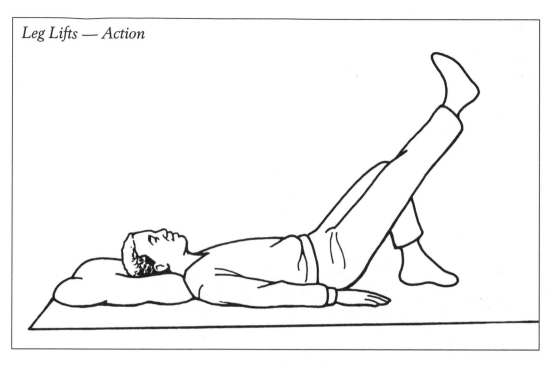

Action.   Exhale and lift your straight leg off the bed to a 45-degree angle to the ceiling. Inhale and release down. Repeat 5–10 times with each leg.

Notes.   Pull in your abdominal muscles to support your back. You may limit the height of the lift for comfort. If there is pain in your hip joint because of orthopedic concerns, metastasis, or joint limitation, please modify or refrain from doing this exercise. Another modification: This exercise can be done starting with both knees bent and feet flat on the bed. Then extend one leg at a time toward the ceiling.

6

Chair Exercises: Beginning to Move

Goal: To prepare your body for standing, maintaining balance, and proper posture. To restore and increase lower and upper body strength.

*T*HE FOLLOWING EXERCISES ARE DESIGNED especially for when you are feeling well enough to get out of bed. Perhaps you have a bit more energy, feel a little more steady on your feet, or even feel a little antsy. You might feel as if you'll go crazy if you stay in bed any longer. You may not want to go out for a mile walk by yourself, but you certainly feel that sitting up won't make you dizzy. When you are ready to be off on your own, you want to make sure that your legs can hold you up and that your arms can reach for the cup on the top shelf of your cabinet. With movements designed to prepare you for these everyday activities, like going to work, you're bound to succeed when you actually try them.

Like the bed exercises, some of the exercises in this section can be done with a partner for added resistance. You can also use light hand-held weights or ankle weights. Before you're up and moving around, which you may be trying intermittently anyway, you'll need to build upper and lower body strength for all the everyday activities you did prior to your treatments. This section helps you do just that. Begin slowly, and as before, you can do the whole section or a little at a time. Increase weights gradually and listen to your body. It knows best.

39

Leg Extensions

Benefits: Quadricep (front of thighs) muscles

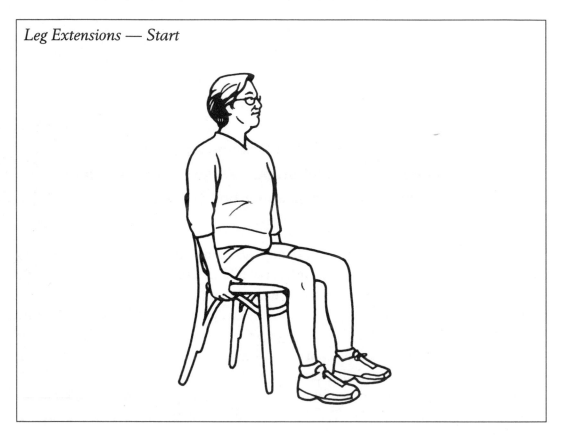

Leg Extensions — Start

Starting position.   Sit on the edge of your chair or bed, keeping your spine long, feet flat on the floor, and your arms down by your side.

Leg Extensions — Action

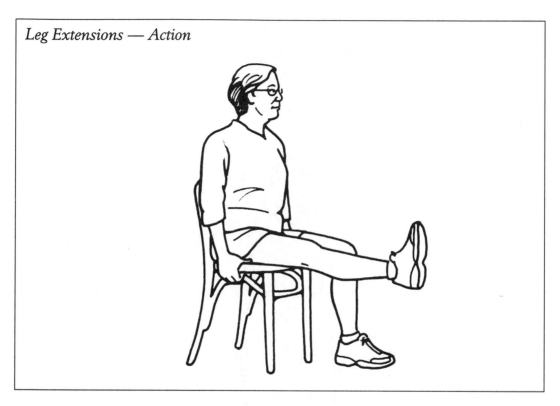

Action.   Exhale and extend one leg; inhale and bring your leg down. Repeat 10 times on each side.

Notes.   You may want to add a few ankle circles to loosen up your ankle joint (to prepare yourself for standing and walking). For added resistance, you can add one- to five-pound ankle weights.

Mid-Back Pull-Backs

Benefits: Rhomboid (mid-back) muscles

Mid-Back Pull-Backs — Start

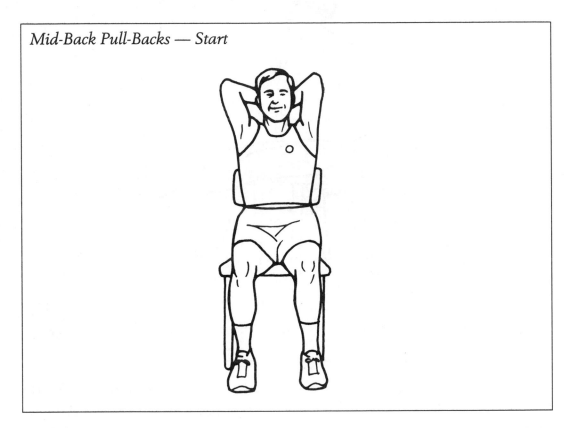

Starting position.　　Sit on the edge of your chair or bed, keeping your spine long and your feet flat on the floor. Bring your palms to the back of your head with your elbows by your ears.

Mid-Back Pull-Backs — Action

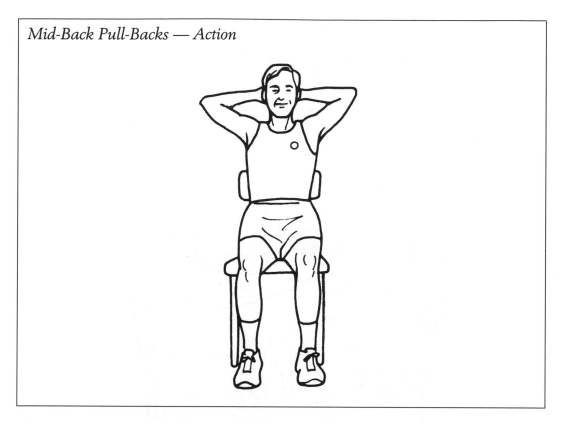

Action. Exhale while bringing your shoulder blades together and your elbows out to the side and hold for 3 counts. Inhale and release. Repeat 10 times.

Notes. Maintain an upright posture by tightening your abdominal muscles. If your shoulder joint or chest area has limited range of motion (ROM) resulting from surgery or if you have a venous port, please modify this exercise for comfort.

Partner Chest Press

Benefits: Pectoral (chest) muscles

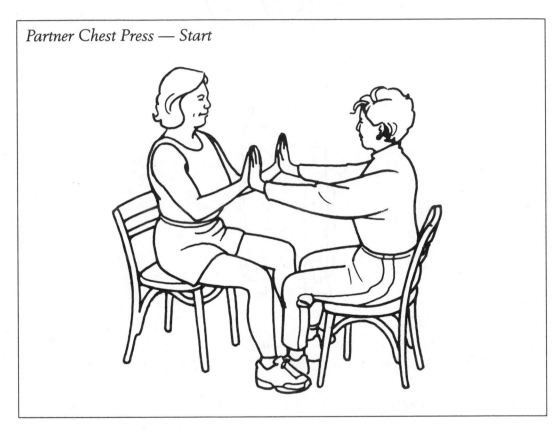

Partner Chest Press — Start

Starting position. Sit on the edge of your chair or bed, keeping your spine long, with feet flat on the floor. Your partner should be sitting in front of you. Place your palms together and slightly bend your elbows.

Partner Chest Press — Action

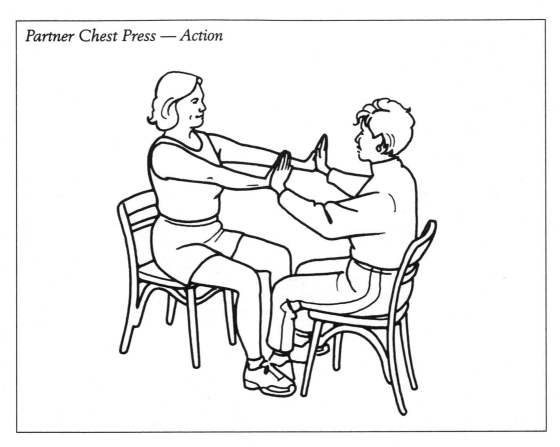

Action. Exhale as you try to push your partner's hands away and hold for 5 counts. Inhale and release to starting position. Repeat 10 times.

Notes. If this position is uncomfortable for you because of limitations in your shoulder and chest area, you can simply clasp both hands together and press together for 5 counts, then release. You can repeat this isometric contraction 5–10 times.

Partner Pull-Backs

Benefits: Rhomboid (mid-back), latissimus dorsi (back), and arm muscles

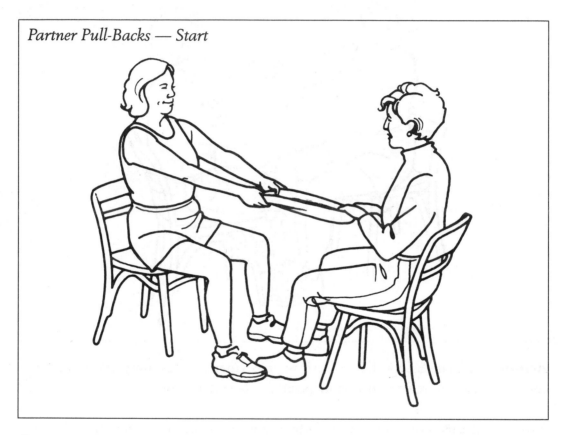

Partner Pull-Backs — Start

Starting position.   Sit on the edge of your chair or bed, keeping your spine long, with feet flat on the floor. With your arms straight out in front of you, hold onto the ends of a towel. Your partner is sitting on a chair in front of you, holding onto the middle of the towel.

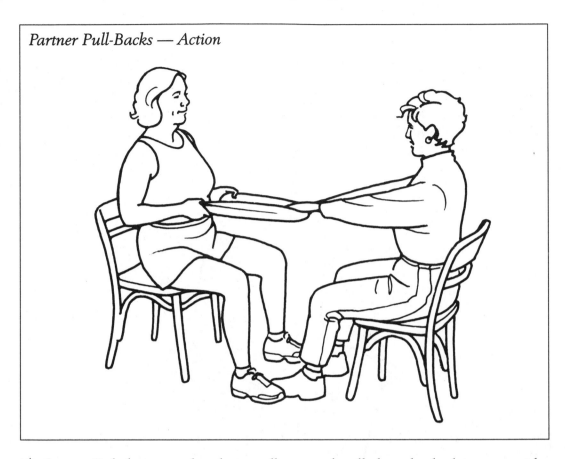

Partner Pull-Backs — Action

Action.   Exhale as you bend your elbows and pull them back along your side, squeezing your shoulder blades together. Your partner should give you some resistance. Inhale and then give your partner some resistance to return to your starting position. It's an exercise for both of you! Repeat 10 times.

Bicep Curls

Benefits: Bicep (front of arm) muscles

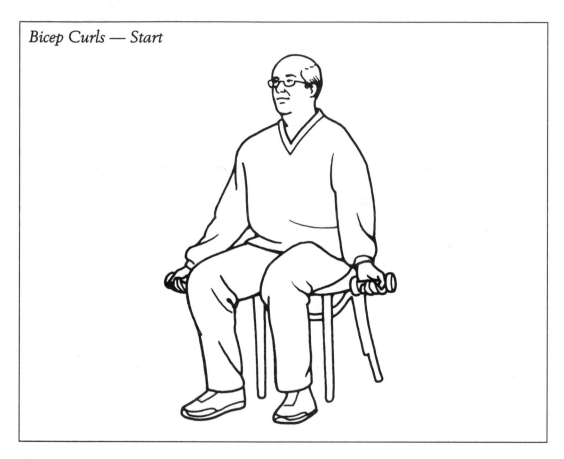

Bicep Curls — Start

Starting position.   Sit on the edge of your chair or bed, keeping your spine long, with feet flat on the floor. Hold your weights with your palms facing forward, elbows along sides.

Bicep Curls — Action

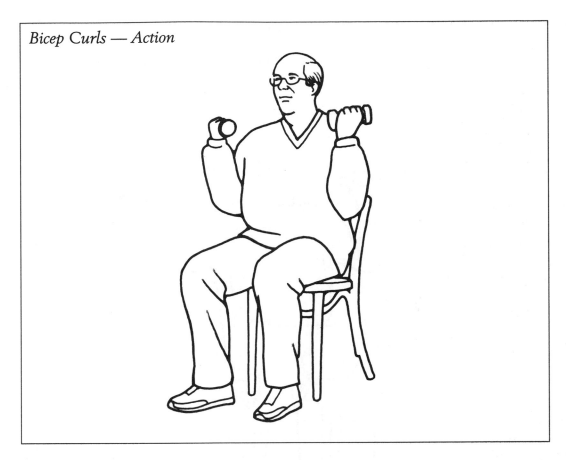

Action. Exhale and bend both elbows, bringing the weights up to your shoulders. Inhale and slowly release down. Repeat 5–10 times.

Notes. This exercise and the following one are for arm strength. If you would like more resistance for an added challenge, try holding between one- and ten-pound hand-held weights, depending on your strength. Begin conservatively with lower weight. When it becomes easy to lift the weight 10 times, increase your weight in one- to two-pound increments for a few weeks.

Overhead Lifts

Benefits: Deltoid (shoulder) muscles

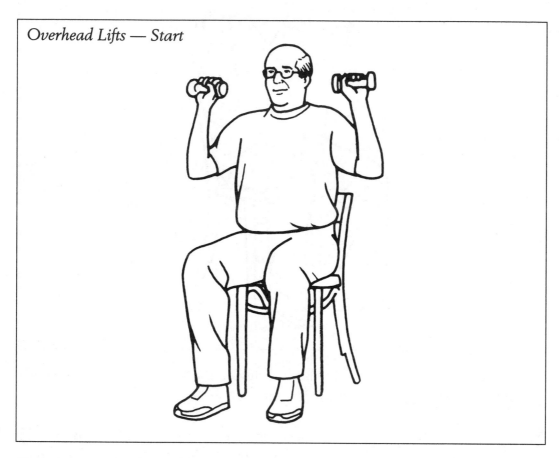

Overhead Lifts — Start

Starting position.   Sit on the edge of your chair or bed, keeping your spine long, with feet flat on the floor. Hold your weights with your palms facing forward, resting the weights on your shoulders.

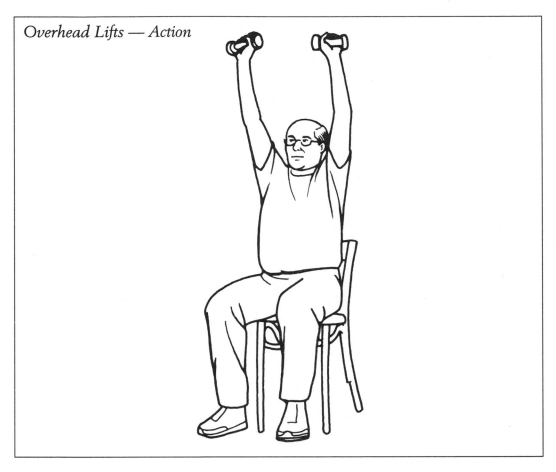

Overhead Lifts — Action

Action.   Exhale and slowly extend your arms straight overhead. Inhale and bend your elbows as you lower the weights to your shoulders.

Notes.   Maintain an upright posture by tightening your abdominal muscles. Repeat 5–10 times. If your shoulder joint has limited range of motion (ROM) because of surgery or a venous port, please modify for comfort by lifting one arm at a time or change the direction of your arms to face each other instead of straight ahead. Another modification: If you feel discomfort in your shoulder area, try to lift light weights with your arms out to the side.

7

Standing Exercises: Walking, Balance, Building Endurance

Goal: Getting back into a routine

*I*F YOU ARE SPENDING MORE TIME OUT OF BED than lying in bed and are back to some of your normal life's work and activities, then this section is for you. To do these exercises, you will need to be able to balance and coordinate your movements. By this time, you are feeling more like the old you. Your routine for treatment has settled in, either for radiation or chemotherapy treatments, or you are a few weeks past surgery. You have fewer limitations and feel that it's time to move forward.

In the following exercises, you can work a bit more independently than before, although you may want a chair for support. Your partner is there if you need the help, mostly for balance, but as for lifting the appropriate weight and maintaining good form, you are on your own. These are basic exercises to support upper and lower body strength. These are known as weight-bearing exercises, which simply means standing on one or two feet to benefit your bones, muscles, and posture. Try to do each exercise at least five times, then you can increase to ten times. If you want added resistance you may add a hand-held weight or an ankle weight for certain exercises.

Stand and Sit

*Benefits: Lower body (quadriceps, hamstrings, gluteus)
muscles and abdominals*

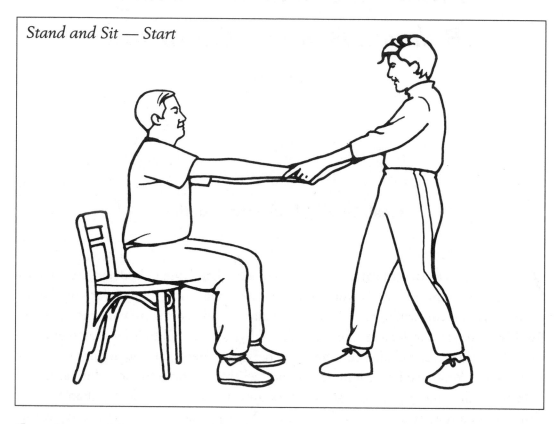

Stand and Sit — Start

Starting position. Sit on the edge of your chair, keeping your spine long, feet flat on the floor, and hands holding onto your partner's hands (your partner is standing in front of you for support).

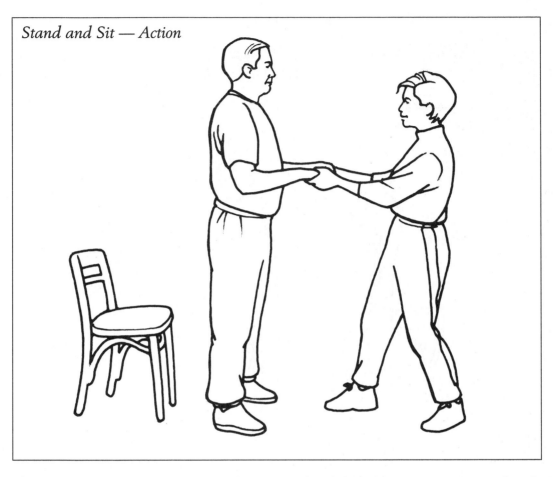

Stand and Sit — Action

Action.   Exhale and rise to standing position while holding your partner's hands only for support. Use your legs for power. Inhale and gently sit back down. Repeat 5–10 times.

Notes.   Keep your knees and feet hip-width apart at all times. Lean forward with weight over your toes as you stand and sit. As you become more comfortable with this exercise, you can try it on your own, with your hands on the chair for leverage or with your arms straight out in front of you.

One-Arm Rows

Benefits: Rhomboid (midback), latissimus dorsi (back),
and bicep (front of arm) muscles

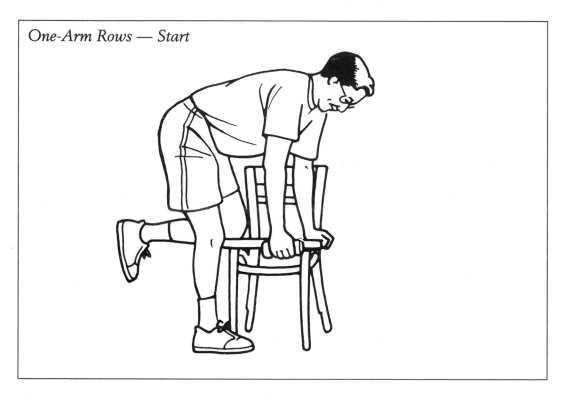

One-Arm Rows — Start

Starting position.   Stand beside a chair. Rest one knee and one hand on the chair. Your back should be parallel to the floor, with your head down. Hold a weight or water bottle in your other hand, extending your arm down.

One-Arm Rows — Action

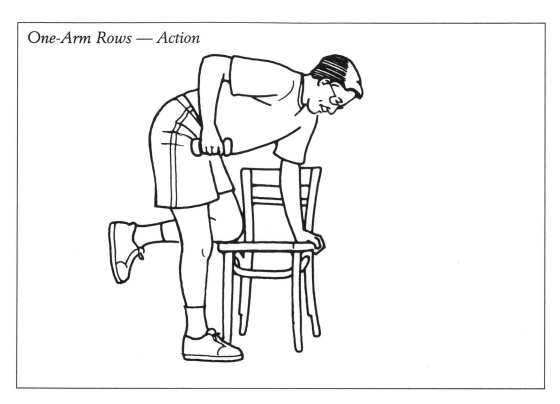

Action. Exhale and bend your elbow, bringing your arm up so your elbow is above your back. Inhale as you bring your arm down. Pull up and down slowly 10 times, then repeat on the other side.

Notes. Use a weight that is comfortable for you to lift up and down 10 times. You can use a small water bottle or a hand-held weight that does not exceed 10 pounds—increase the weight slowly and wisely. Use your back muscles for the lift (your shoulder blade should move with the action). For an added stretch before the exercise, you can hold onto the weight with your arm straight down to the floor and move your arm in small circles in each direction. Lifting heavy weight is not recommended for those at risk of lymphedema.

Standing Wall Push-Ups

Benefits: Pectoral (chest), tricep (back of arm) muscles

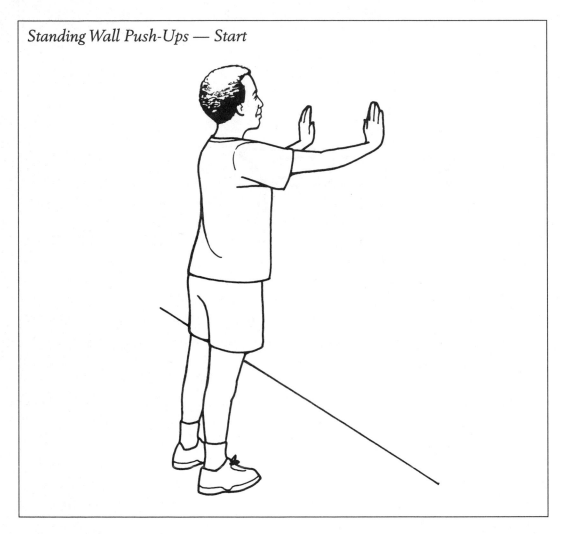

Standing Wall Push-Ups — Start

Starting position.   Standing, place both hands on the wall, with arms straight and fingertips facing up.

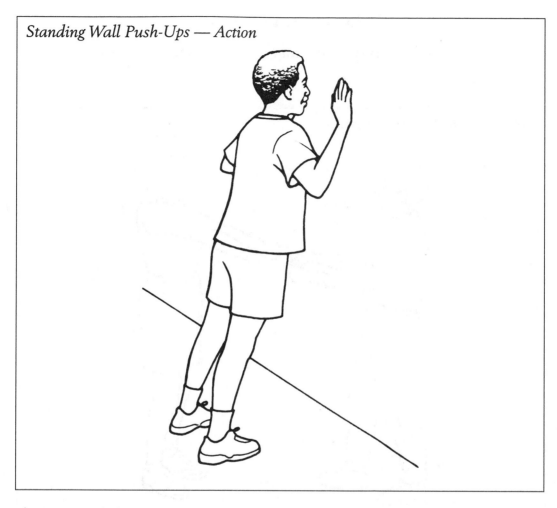

Standing Wall Push-Ups — Action

Action.   Inhale and bend your elbows as you lean into the wall. Exhale and push out, so your arms straighten. Repeat 10 times.

Notes.   For added stretch and ROM at shoulder joint, simply face the wall and crawl your fingers up the wall as far as you can, then crawl down. This exercise can also be done facing the wall sideways and crawling up the wall with one palm facing up. This may be familiar to those recovering from breast surgery.

Balance with Partner

Benefits: Balance and sensory awareness

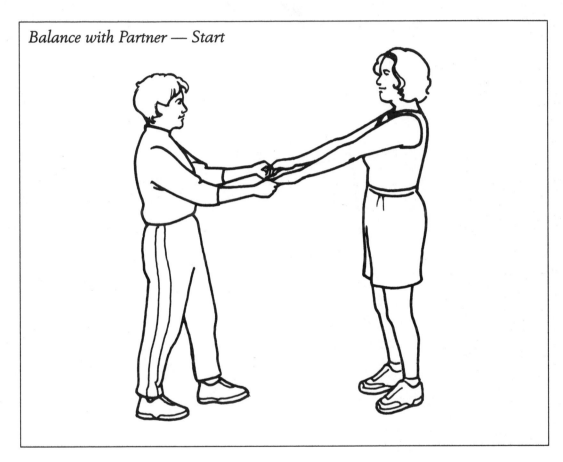

Balance with Partner — Start

Starting position.   Stand in front of your partner holding onto their hands.

Balance with Partner — Action

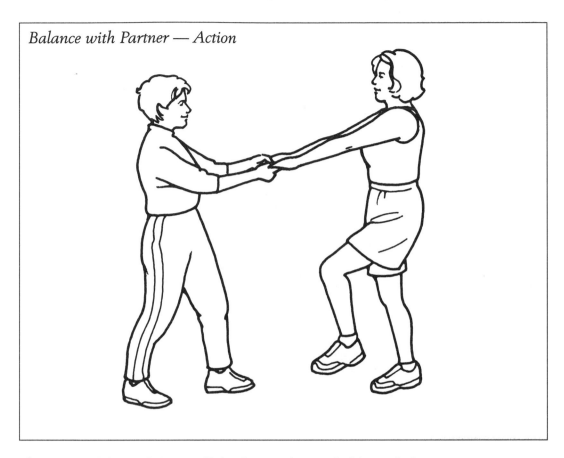

Action. Pick one foot up off the floor and try to hold your balance up to 10 counts. Breathe normally throughout. Alternate legs and repeat 4 times.

Notes. As you become more comfortable in your balance, let go of your partner's hands to try it by yourself. Your partner should be there to help at any time.

Knee Lifts

Benefits: Psoas (hip flexor) muscles and balance

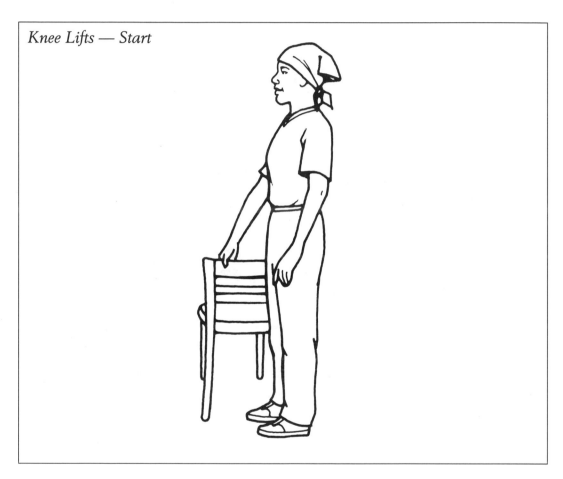

Knee Lifts — Start

Starting position.   Stand in back of your chair and turn to the side.

Knee Lifts — Action

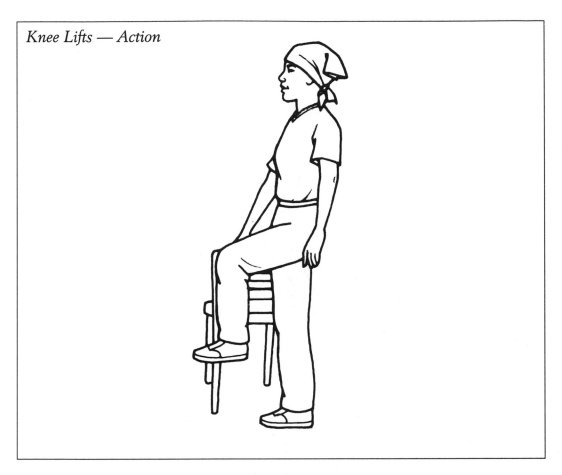

Action. Exhale and bend one knee, lifting it off the floor to a comfortable height. Inhale and release down. Alternate legs. Repeat 10 times.

Hamstring Curls

Benefits: Hamstring (back of leg) muscles

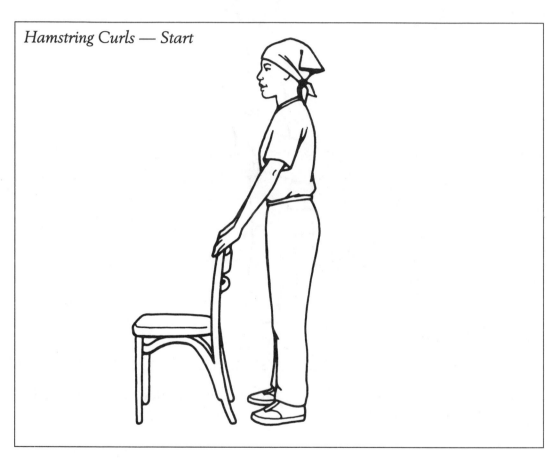

Hamstring Curls — Start

Starting position.   Stand with both legs hip-width apart and place both hands against the wall or behind a chair for balance.

Hamstring Curls — Action

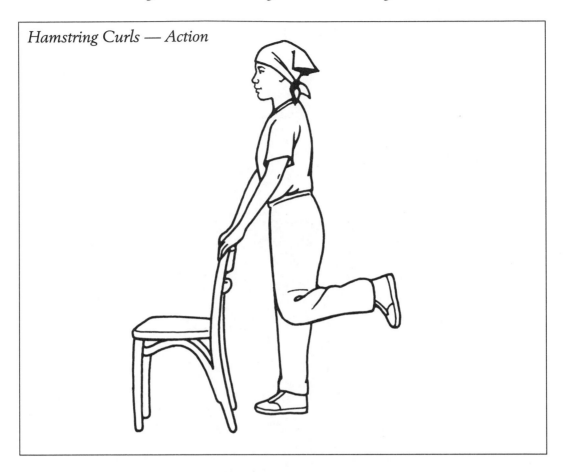

Action.   Exhale and bend at the knee, bringing your heel up to your buttocks. Inhale while slowly releasing down. Repeat 10 times. Then change to the other side.

Notes.   Keep your abdomen firm (imagine pulling your belly button toward your spine) to avoid arching your lower back, and keep your knees together. For added resistance you can add one- to five-pound ankle weights.

8

Stretching

〜

**The following stretches can be done
lying in a bed, on the floor, or standing. Remember,
stretching is recommended during all stages of treatment.**

STRETCHING IS A WONDERFUL WAY TO GET IN TOUCH with the intimate connection between your body and your mind. When you settle down to stretch, you can feel the areas that are tight from the physical and emotional stress of your day.

If you breathe deeply and relax into your stretching exercises, you will find yourself more flexible mentally as well as physically. Stretching can open up a sense of being calm and centered.

There are many different ways to stretch a muscle and loosen up stiff areas of your body. In *The Healing Power of Movement* we use static stretching. This involves slowly lengthening a muscle to the point of tension, then holding the position for about twenty seconds. With static stretching there is less chance of stretching beyond your limits and risking injury or soreness.

Lower Back Stretch

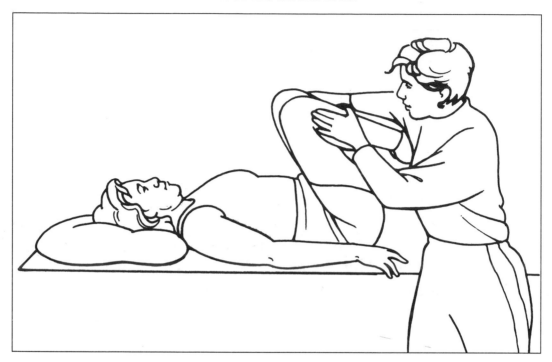

Lower Back Stretch

Lie on your back with both knees bent and your feet flat on the floor or bed. One at a time, bring your knees into your chest. Your partner can lightly press your knees into your chest. Hold for twenty seconds and then release. If you have knee concerns, your partner can hold onto you under your knees. You should feel a stretch in your lower back. Communicate; let your partner know if he or she is pressing enough or not enough. Lacking a partner, you can hold your knees to your chest on your own.

Hamstring Stretch

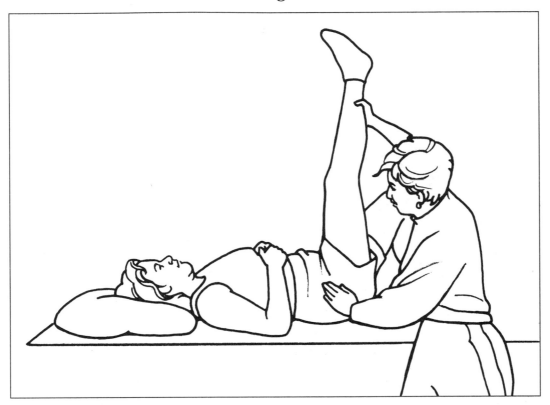

Hamstring Stretch

Lie on your back with both knees bent and your feet flat on the floor or bed. Bring one knee into your chest, then extend the leg straight up, keeping both hips down. Your partner can help you lift your leg up toward the ceiling. Once your leg is extended straight and your foot is up toward the ceiling, hold that position for twenty seconds—your partner can hold it there for you. Gently release and repeat with the other leg. If you lack a partner, you can simply hold onto your straight leg with your hands holding onto your thigh.

Back Stretch with Twist

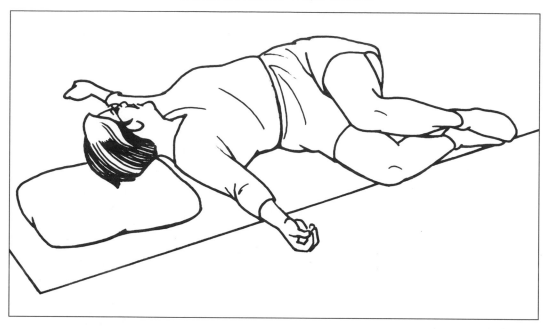

Back Stretch with Twist

Lie on your back with both knees bent and your feet flat on the floor or bed. One at a time, bring your knees into your chest. Let both knees gently fall over to one side and look in the opposite direction. You can ask your partner to guide you and help you relax and breathe deeply into this stretch. Breathe into this stretch for about twenty to thirty seconds, then switch to the other side.

If you have been diagnosed with osteoporosis, have any back conditions that prevent you from twisting, or if you are sensitive on one side owing to treatment, please refrain from doing this stretch.

Back Release and Chest Stretch

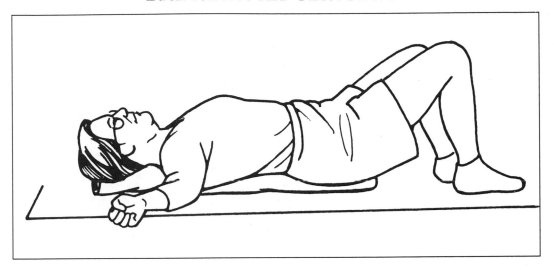

Back Release and Chest Stretch

Lie on a rolled towel placed lengthwise under your spine with your head resting on the towel. Open your arms out to the side with the palms up. Your knees can be bent with both feet flat on the floor or both legs can be extended straight down, depending on what is most comfortable. Breathe deeply in this position. Hold for twenty to thirty seconds. This exercise is recommended to relieve tension and tightness in the chest, upper back, and shoulder areas.

Quadriceps Stretch

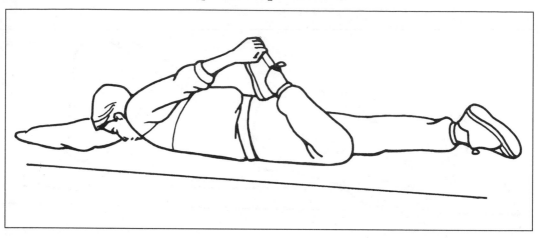

Quadriceps Stretch

Lie on your stomach with your face down. Bend one knee behind you and grab your foot. Bring your heel toward your buttocks, as close as possible without straining, breathing deeply. Hold for twenty seconds. Slowly release down. Repeat with other leg. For added comfort for your lower back, place a pillow under your stomach. This exercise can be modified to a standing position holding onto a wall or chair for balance.

If it is necessary, your partner can help you hold onto your foot for the stretch.

Standing Chest Stretch

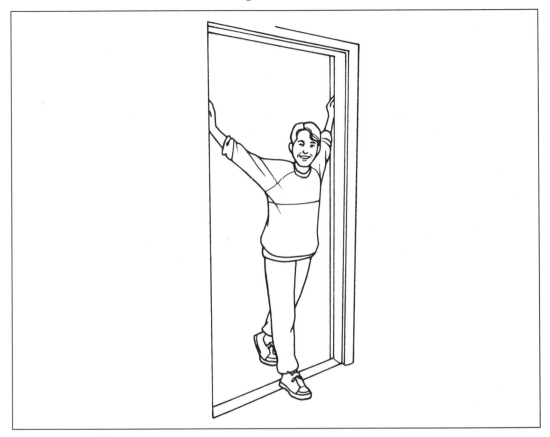

Standing Chest Stretch

Stand in a doorway and hold onto the sides with your elbows bent at 90-degree angles. Step forward with one leg, as if you're walking into the room, so that your elbows are slightly behind you and your chest is open. Hold for 20 seconds.

Notes. If you have a port in your chest area, this stretch is not recommended if it is uncomfortable. If you feel tightness in the chest owing to surgery, stretch the chest area gently after getting your physician's approval. This exercise can also be done in a corner of the room bending your elbows at 90-degree angles and leaning into the corner.

9

Physical Activity Chart

$\mathcal{F}$OLLOWING IS AN ACTIVITY CHART I PUT TOGETHER to give an idea of the type of physical exercise you might consider for different stages and types of cancer treatment. The left-hand column details the system affected. The middle columns provide information about physical concerns and symptoms you may experience following the different types of treatments, and the right-hand column gives suggestions for physical activities.

Cancer Treatment Strategies and Physical Activity Recommendations

Surgery (localized)

System	Concerns	Physical Activity Recommendation
Joint/muscle limitation	Incision areas, muscles cut during surgery, part or all of muscle may be removed. In reconstruction, may have tightness and soreness in area.	• Prior to surgery, maintain muscle strength to help in recovery. Will be asked to get out of bed shortly after surgery. • Prior to surgery, stretch the area that will be affected to help in flexibility. • Begin limited (bed exercises) program 1–2 weeks postsurgery, as per physician.
Lymphatic system Impairment of lymph system	If lymph nodes are removed, there may be some short- and long-term concerns regarding lymphedema and infection.	• Slow, progressive exercise, increasing ROM, facilitate draining with pumping action, compression (area where lymph nodes were taken), to begin program as per physician. • May incorporate diaphragmatic breathing, passive exercise, isometrics (contract/release) within a few days postsurgery.

Neurological	Neuropathy; numbness, loss of sensation around incision or nerve damage from incision.	• Moderate movement in limbs to facilitate mobility. • Breathing techniques and relaxation may help in sensory awareness. • Focus on various balancing exercises for stability.

Chemotherapy (systemic)

System	Side Effects	Symptoms	Physical Activity Recommendation
Cardiovascular	Cardiomyopathy Pulmonary restrictions	Heart palpitations Arrhythmias Shortness of breath Leg swelling Exhaustion Shift in blood pressure Dizziness	• Your aerobic capacity may be compromised; therefore, intermittent (stop and start) exercise is recommended. • Type of activity can vary—walking/cycling/swimming • Begin the following exercise program in a slow, progressive manner. • When changing body positions for exercises from a sitting or lying position to a standing position, move slowly to decrease dizziness and dramatic shifts in blood pressure. • With prolonged bed rest, blood pressure, pulmonary function, and bone density may be compromised, therefore it is recommended to get out of bed and move around.
	Decrease in RBCs	Anemia Fatigue	• Your aerobic capacity may be compromised; therefore, intermittent (stop and start) exercise is recommended. • Heart rate during activity should be low to moderate (40–60 percent of maximum heart rate—Max = rate × 220-age). • Begin exercise when appropriate in a slow, progressive manner. • Maintain proper breathing patterns with given exercise.
	Decrease in WBCs	Susceptibility to infection Fatigue	• It is recommended to partake in non-contact sports or activities to decrease risk of injury. • Before and after using equipment, wash your hands. • Begin exercise when appropriate in a slow, progressive manner.

Cardiovascular *(continued)*	Low platelet count	Risk of bleeding Bruising	• Avoid contact sports and other activities that might result in cuts or bruising.
Neurological	Peripheral neuropathy	A tingling, burning, weakness, or numbness in the hands and/or feet. Other nerve-related symptoms include loss of balance, clumsiness, difficulty picking up objects and buttoning clothing, walking problems, jaw pain, hearing loss, stomach pain, and constipation.	• Maintain movement at the extremities (fingers, toes). Wiggle your fingers and toes a few times a day. • If your sense of balance is affected, you can avoid falls by moving carefully, using handrails when going up or down stairs, and using bath mats in the bathtub or shower. • Practice balancing exercises and focus on leg exercises along with maintaining core (torso) stability.
Gastro-intestinal	Nausea, vomiting Mucositis Loss of appetite Constipation Diarrhea	May limit ability to eat well and absorb needed nutrients.	• With decreased energy, it may be difficult to sustain activity. Instead, intermittent activity is recommended. • Activity for a prolonged period of time may be uncomfortable if diarrhea is a concern. • Full-body activity may aid in digestion and removal of waste if constipation is a concern.
Other	Hair loss Nail thinning/loss Skin irritation	Redness, itching, peeling, dryness, and acne. Your nails may become darkened, brittle, or cracked. They also may develop vertical lines or bands. Some people report feeling as though they have the flu a few hours to a few days after chemotherapy. Flulike symptoms—muscle aches, headache, tiredness, nausea, slight fever, chills, and poor appetite—may last from 1–3 days.	• In cool weather use head covering to maintain body temperature. • Use sunscreen when outside for walking or cycling. • Use caution when handling weights or exercise equipment if nail thinning or breaking is a concern. • Skin irritation should not affect walking, cycling, or swimming abilities, however, chlorinated pools may irritate the skin. • With flulike symptoms, work within your capabilities at this time.

| Women | Anticancer drugs may damage the ovaries and reduce the amount of hormones they produce. As a result, some women find that their menstrual periods become irregular or stop completely while they are receiving chemotherapy. | The hormonal effects of chemotherapy also may cause menopauselike symptoms such as hot flashes and itching, burning, or dryness of vaginal tissues. | • Maintain physical activity to maintain muscle mass and enhance cardiorespiratory conditioning.
• Perform weight-bearing activity to promote bone health (any activity with your feet on the ground, such as walking, stair climbing, dancing).
• Focus on torso strengthening and back, chest, and abdominal muscles. Promote good posture.
• Relaxation techniques may help in coping with hot flashes and other menopauselike symptoms. |

Radiation

System	Side Effects	Symptoms	Physical Activity Recommendation
Localized	Head and neck: hypothyroidism, esophagus, mucositis Chest: cardiac toxicity Pelvic area: vaginal complications, bladder and gastrointestinal issues, hematuria	The body uses energy to heal itself. Any symptoms are mostly felt after a few weeks of radiation therapy. In some cases, onset of side effects may not happen until a few years later.	• Your aerobic capacity may be compromised; therefore, intermittent (stop and start) exercise is recommended. • Heart rate during activity should be low to moderate (40–60 percent of maximum heart rate—max = rate × 220-age) for cardiac protection. • Begin exercise when appropriate in a slow, progressive manner. You may want to stay away from any impact or jarring activity for bladder concerns. • Maintain proper breathing patterns with any given exercise. • Depending on the site radiated, site-specific exercise may feel difficult. Range of motion at the area may feel limited. Therefore, gently move the area to increase mobility.
Skin	Short-term changes in skin appearance Long-term changes (6–10 months) Thickening of the skin	Itchy, dry, flushed, warm, uncomfortable	• Moisturize dry skin area, as approved by physician, and when handling exercise equipment to protect skin from cracking. • Area of skin that is radiated may become tight and limit the range of motion. Work progressively to maintain mobility.

System	Side Effects		Physical Activity Recommendation
Skin (*continued*)			• Perform exercise program in a well-ventilated room to help prevent overheating. Drinking plenty of water is recommended. • Wear loose-fitting clothes to decrease skin irritation.
Lymphatic	May initiate onset of lymphedema by scar formation or skin burn.	Lymphedema	• Enhance lymphatic circulation with diaphragmatic breathing. • Isometric, hand-squeezing, or pumping exercises. • Use light weights for upper body strengthening in a progressive manner.

Transplant (systemic)

System	Side Effects	Physical Activity Recommendation
Bone marrow/stem cell transplant	Affects WBC/RBC platelets	• Start program 3–4 weeks posttransplant, with the bed, chair, and standing program or as recommended by your physician. • May perform intermittent walking or stationary cycling. • Modify movement if sore from biopsy area.

10

Perspective

I AM ALWAYS LEARNING FROM THE ATTITUDES of our clients, and most recently I have been struck by the words of a woman I started working with seven months before she was diagnosed with breast cancer. Sandy started working out with Solo Fitness to get a consistent workout with a motivated trainer who would also help her lose weight. Then she received the cancer diagnosis. Sandy anticipated the worst, having heard stories of the nausea and exhaustion she would likely experience and the limitations to her life. She decided to do all she could to help herself handle the cancer therapy in a healthy and proactive way.

Today Sandy has made it through chemotherapy as well as lat flap reconstructive surgery, during which the surgeon pulled part of her back muscle to the front to fill in where there used to be breast tissue. In addition, however, Sandy has seen a psychoanalyst, an acupuncturist, and a nutritionist. She maintained her workouts with Solo Fitness and is considering starting yoga lessons. She thanks her doctor for being progressive enough to understand that her treatment strategy can include all these other aspects. Unlike some stories she has heard, Sandy was not told to just go home and deal with the effects of chemotherapy on her own.

I can only describe Sandy's reaction to her cancer diagnosis as being suddenly energized to organize her life. She now takes time to figure out all of her nutrition requirements, when and how often to take her various botanicals, and to make appointments with her complementary practitioners in addition to maintaining her regimen of chemotherapy every three weeks for six cycles and continuing to work.

Sandy is open about her ordeal. "Now that I'm bald," she said to me early on in her treatments, "I have my wig ready to use when I need it. Otherwise, I have baseball caps in every color to match my outfits." She hasn't been overly fatigued at one point or the other during her treatment as she expected and was told she would be. "Must be that I'm eating more frequently during the day, exercising, and regenerating with a massage. What else would it be?"

As far as Sandy's workouts with me, we have almost followed our original plan except to modify certain exercises because of limited range of motion around the shoulder and upper back area, or during the periods right after her chemotherapy when she takes a drug to boost the immune system that leaves her with muscle stiffness and an overall malaise. We have changed the amount of weight she lifts, the number of repetitions of her exercises, and the intensity of her stretching, but she still exclaims over the feeling of exhilaration she gets when she moves her body. To still have control over her body and to be able to systematically exercise has made a physical and mental difference in Sandy's cancer therapy.

After all she went through in the first three months, Sandy surprised me when she looked at me and said, "I feel healthier now with cancer than before I was diagnosed." That's how I keep learning from my clients.

Jack has made me realize something else: the value of keeping life in perspective. Since 1998, Jack has gone through two bouts of Hodgkin's lymphoma with treatment including stem cell transplant and radiation. For two years of our workouts my challenge was to constantly modify exercises for whatever his level of fitness was. Sometimes he was overwhelmed with fatigue and we had to take a pause, or he became nauseated and had to leave the room, or the range of motion of his shoulder joint was limited because of his implanted port. For some periods of time Jack was so weakened by his cancer treatments that he could barely move. Even then, he somehow amassed the energy to write in a journal. Throughout the years of fighting cancer, Jack was mostly consistent in doing some sort of exercise three days a week and tried to report to his office daily to keep a feeling of normalcy in his days.

Now it's been at least two years since Jack was diagnosed with cancer and our workouts have returned to normal. Jack is back to the usual aches and pains that he had prior to cancer. His lower back frequently bothers him, and he has since been diagnosed with a herniated disc. After all Jack has been through, however, the pain of an aching back is hardly a life-threatening problem. These days he barely mentions what used to be a cause for complaint. It's all a matter of perspective.

Working with our clients from the day of diagnosis through their last day of treatment has certainly been a ride. Sometimes the ride has progressed full steam ahead, and other times stalled in the station. The underlying thought many times has been, this too will pass. And it has. When our clients get back to regular daily activities that they used to take for granted, they view their days through different eyes. Sometimes it's a pause on the way to work to look at the scenery or to smile at a neighbor on the bus or to say thank-you to a coworker. The little moments don't go by without notice.

Life has many lessons for us, but none greater than when one is faced with a potentially terminal illness. No one comes through cancer treatment without being changed, and that's good. I have found the biggest change in our clients to be that they are more optimistic. The healing power of movement has changed not only their muscles but their lives.

Many years ago when I was a dance major in college, I took a dance composition class during which we were expected to choreograph our own pieces. As it turned out, a few weeks into the semester I tore the left anterior cruciate ligament in my knee and was unable to dance for the rest of the semester. Not wanting to drop the class, I decided I could still choreograph a piece for another group of dancers. Since I was unable to put any weight on my left leg, I choreographed a piece titled "For a Bad Left Knee," in which the dancer uses one healthy leg and two healthy arms. It turned out to be quite a creative dance. It was impossible for me to accept the fact that I couldn't dance; movement has always been the way I express myself best and the way I stay comfortable in my own body. I felt that if I had to live with the impairment, at least I could move the parts of me that still worked. Of course, injuring a knee is a far cry from a cancer diagnosis, but it reminds me of the perceived limitations we can have when we are dealt a physical blow.

Today the medical profession calls cancer a chronic disease. The National Cancer Institute estimates that about 8.2 million Americans are living with cancer in various stages of treatment, remission, and cure. Just as they're changing their perception of the disease, health professionals are starting to change their ideas about how much activity a cancer patient can handle while in treatment or soon after.

My desire is that you are inspired by this book to remain active, no matter how impaired you may be from fighting cancer. My desire is that you find a way to choreograph your own dance and to move the parts of you that still work.

Bibliography

ACSM's Guidelines for Exercise Testing and Prescription, 4th and 5th eds. Media, Pa.: Lea and Febiger, 1991; Williams and Wilkens, 1995.

Brennan, M., and L. Miller. "Overview of Treatment Options and Review of the Current Role and Use of Compression Garments, Intermittent Pumps, and Exercise in the Management of Lymphedema." *Cancer* 83, no. 12 (1998): 2821–2827.

CDC, National Center for Chronic Disease Prevention and Health Promotion. "President's Council on Physical Fitness and Sports: Physical Activity and Health; A Report of the Surgeon General." Pittsburg, Pa.: CDC, 1996.

Courneya, K. S., and C. M. Friedenreich. "Physical Exercise and Quality of Life Following Cancer Diagnosis: A Literature Review." *Annals of Behavioral Medicine* 21, no. 2 (spring 1999): 171–179.

_____. "Determinants of Exercise During Colorectal Cancer Treatment: An Application of the Theory of Planned Behavior." *ONF* 24, no. 10 (1997): 1715–1723.

Courneya, K. S., J. R. Mackey, and L. W. Jones. "Coping with Cancer: Can Exercise Help?" *Physician and Sportsmedicine* 28, no. 5 (May 2000).

Cunningham, B. A., G. Morris, C. Cheney, N. Buergel, S. N. Acker, and P. Lenssen. "Effects of Resistive Exercise on Skeletal Muscle in Marrow Transplant Recipients Receiving Total Parenteral Nutrition." *Journal of Parenteral and Enteral Nutrition* 10, no. 6 (1986): 558–563.

Daneryd, P., E. Svanberg, U. Körner, E. Lindholm, R. Sandström, H. Breuinge, C. Pettersson, I. Bosaeus, and K. Lundholm. "Protection of Metabolic and Exercise

Capacity in Unselected Weight-Losing Cancer Patients Following Treatment with Recombinant Erythropoietin: A Randomized Prospective Study." *Cancer Research* 58 (1998): 5374–5379.

Decker, W. A., J. Turner-McGlade, and K. M. Fehir. "Psychosocial Aspects and the Physiological Effects of a Cardiopulmonary Exercise Program in Patients Undergoing Bone Marrow Transplantation (BMT) for Acute Leukemia (AL)." *Transplantation Proceedings* 21, no. 1 (February 1989): 3068–3069.

Dimeo, F., H. Bertz, J. Finke, S. Fetscher, R. Mertelsmann, and J. Keul. "An Aerobic Exercise Program for Patients with Haematological Malignancies after Bone Marrow Transplantation." *Bone Marrow Transplantation* 18 (1996): 1157–1160.

Dimeo, F., S. Fetscher, W. Lange, R. Mertelsmann, and J. Keul. "Effects of Aerobic Exercise on the Physical Performance and Incidence of Treatment-Related Complications After High-Dose Chemotherapy." *Blood* 90, no. 9 (1997): 3390–3394.

Dimeo, F., B. G. Rumberger, and J. Keul. "Aerobic Exercise as Therapy for Cancer Fatigue." *Medicine and Science in Sports and Exercise* 30, no. 4 (1998): 475–478.

Dimeo, F., M. Tilmann, H. Bertz, L. Kanz, R. Mertelsmann, and J. Keul. "Aerobic Exercise in the Rehabilitation of Cancer Patients after High-Dose Chemotherapy and Autologous Peripheral Stem Cell Transplantation." *Cancer* 79, no. 9 (1997): 1717–1722.

Gerhardsson de Verdier, M. "Physical Activity in the Prevention and Management of Cancer." *World Review of Nutrition and Diet* 82 (1997): 240–249.

Goodfrey, C. M. "'Yes' to Exercise for Breast Cancer Survivors." *JAMC* (Canadian Medical Association Journal) 159, no. 11 (December 1, 1998).

Graydon, J., N. Bubela, and D. Irvine. "Fatigue-Reducing Strategies Used by Patients Receiving Treatment for Cancer." *Cancer Nursing* 18, no. 1 (1995): 23–28.

Hoffman, L. B., and A. Weil Bell. *Better Than Ever: The 4-Week Workout Program for Women Over 40.* Chicago: Contemporary Books, 1997.

Hoffman-Goetz, T., B. MacNeil, Y. Arumugam, and J. Randall Simpson. "Differential Effects of Exercise and Housing Condition on Murine Natural Killer Cell Activity and Tumor Growth." *International Journal of Sports Medicine* 13, no. 2 (1992): 167–171.

Jain, B., A. A. Floreani, J. R. Anderson, J. M. Vose, R. A. Robbins, S. I. Rennard, and J. H. Sisson. "Cardiopulmonary Function and Autologous Bone Marrow Transplantation: Results and Predictive Value for Respiratory Failure and Mortality." *Bone Marrow Transplantation* 17 (1996): 561–568.

Lappe, J. M., and S. T. Tinley. "Prevention of Osteoporosis in Women Treated for Hereditary Breast and Ovarian Carcinoma—A Need That Is Overlooked." *Cancer* 83, no. 5 (September 1, 1998): 830–834.

MacVicar M., M. Winningham, and J. Nickel. "Effects of Aerobic Interval Training on Cancer Patients' Functional Capacity." *Nursing Research* 38, no. 6 (1989): 348–351.

McKay, J., and N. Hirano. *The Chemotherapy and Radiation Therapy Survival Guide.* Oakland, Calif.: New Harbinger Publications, 1998.

McTiernan, A., C. Ulrich, C. Kumai, D. Beam, R. Schwartz, J. Mahloch, R. Hastings, J. Gralow, and J. Potter. "Anthropometric and Hormone Effects of an Eight-Week Exercise-Diet Intervention in Breast Cancer Patients: Results of a Pilot Study." *Cancer Epidemiology, Biomarkers and Prevention* 7 (1998): 477–481.

McTiernan, A., C. Ulrich, S. Slate, and J. Potter. "Physical Activity and Cancer Etiology: Associations and Mechanisms." *Cancer Causes and Control* 9 (1998): 487–509.

Mock, V., M. Burke Barton, and P. Sheehan. "A Nursing Rehabilitation Program for Women with Breast Cancer Receiving Adjuvant Chemotherapy." *Oncology Nurses Forum* 21, no. 5 (1994): 899–907.

Mock, V., K. H. Dow, C. J. Meares, P. M. Grimm, J. A. Dienemann, M. E. Haisfield-Wolf, W. Quitasol, S. Mitchell, A. Chakravarthy, and I. Gage. "Effects of Exercise on Fatigue, Physical Functioning, and Emotional Distress During Radiation Therapy for Breast Cancer." *Oncology Nurses Forum* 24, no. 6 (1997): 991–1000.

Mooed, M. A. "Emphasizing and Promoting Overall Health and Nontraditional Treatments after a Prostate Cancer Diagnosis." *Seminars in Urologic Oncology* 17, no. 2 (May 1999): 119–124.

Nieman, D. C. "Exercise Immunology: Practical Applications." *International Journal of Sports Medicine* 18, suppl. 1 (1997): S91–100.

Nieman, D. C., V. D. Cook, D. A. Henson, J. Suttles, W. J. Rejeski, P. M. Ribisl, O. R. Fagoaga, and S. L. Nehlsen-Cannarella. "Moderate Exercise Training and Natural Killer Cell Cytotoxic Activity in Breast Cancer Patients." *International Journal of Sports Medicine* 16 (1995): 334–337.

Pedersen, B. K., and H. Bruunsgaard. "How Physical Exercise Influences the Establishment of Infections." *Sports Medicine* 19, no. 6 (1995): 393–400.

Peters, C., H. Lötzerich, B. Niemeier, K. Schüle, and G. Uhlenbruch. "Influence of a Moderate Exercise Training on Natural Killer Cytotoxicity and Personality Traits in Cancer Patients." *Anticancer Research* 14 (1994): 1033–1036.

Rhind, S. G., G. A. Gannon, M. Suzui, R. J. Shephard, and P. N. Shek. "Indomethacin Inhibits Circulating PGE2 and Reverses Postexercise Suppression of Natural Killer Cell Activity." *American Journal of Physiology* 276, no. 5, pt.2 (1999): R1496–1505.

Rinehart-Ayres, M. E. "Conservative Approaches to Lymphedema Treatment." *Cancer Supplement* 83, no. 12 (December 15, 1998): 2828–2832.

Risberg, T, E. Wist, and R. M. Bremnes. "Patients' Opinion and Use of Nonproven Therapies Related to Their View on Cancer Aetiology." *Anticancer Research* 18 (1998): 499–506.

Schwartz, A. "Patterns of Exercise and Fatigue in Physically Active Cancer Survivors." *Oncology Nurses Forum* 25, no. 3 (1998): 485–491.

Segar, M. L., V. L. Katch, R. S. Roth, A. W. Garcia, T. I. Portner, S. G. Glickman, S. Haslanger, and E. G. Wilkins. "The Effects of Aerobic Exercise on Self-Esteem and Depressive and Anxiety Symptoms among Breast Cancer Survivors." *Oncology Nurses Forum* 25, no.1 (1998): 107–113.

Shephard, R. J. "Physical Activity and Cancer." *International Journal of Sports Medicine* 11 (1990): 413–420.

Smith, S. L. "Physical Exercise as an Oncology Nursing Intervention to Enhance Quality of Life." *Oncology Nurses Forum* 23, no. 5 (1996): 771–778.

Stoll, B. A. "Diet and Exercise Regimens to Improve Breast Carcinoma Prognosis." *CANCER* 78, no. 12 (1996): 2465–2470.

Van Mieghem, W., and M. Demedts. "Cardiopulmonary Function after Lobectomy or Pneumonectomy for Pulmonary Neoplasm." *Respiratory Medicine* 83 (1989): 199–206.

Winningham, M. L. "Walking Program for People with Cancer—Getting Started." *Cancer Nursing* 14, no. 5 (1991): 270–276.

Woods, J. A. "Exercise and Resistance to Neoplasia." *Canadian Journal of Physiology and Pharmacology* 76 (1998): 581–588.

Zanker, K. S., and R. Kroezek. "Looking Along the Track of the Psychoneuroimmunologic Axis for Missing Links in Cancer Progression." *International Journal of Sports Medicine* 12 Suppl. 1 (1991): S58–62.

Acknowledgments

The Healing Power of Movement developed from the day-to-day experiences of working with individuals with cancer. We moved through and looked back on this experience with humility together. As I learned from the beginning with Solo Fitness, projects are anything but solo. It is with much gratitude that I thank the following individuals who were the voices in these pages.

To our clients who have survived their battles: You have taught me, moved me, and provoked me to better understand the wants of your body, the determination of self, and your positive attitude. A special appreciation for sharing your private experiences in a public manner.

To the Solo Fitness staff, a huge thank-you for your encouragement and patience during this endeavor. Your commitment to combine physical activity with a balanced and healthy life for our clients is exceptional.

I would individually like to thank Kathy Cole for your helpful hints in the book development and for working with our clients while giving special attention to their needs, patience with their progress, and an encouraging hand and smile to boot. I thank Joan Pagano for her shared expertise in the physiology of cancer treatment, and critical eye working with breast cancer survivors. Thanks to Ali Martin for loaning her perfect form and figure for the exercise illustrations. I thank the staff at Miracle House, who were open to the idea of the exercise program being available to their clients during their stay in New York City while receiving treatment.

Many thanks to the experts who shared their encouraging words and support for this book. Dr. Fernando Dimeo, Department of Sports Medicine, Free University, Berlin; Dr. Stephen Nimer, head, Division of Hematologic Oncology and chief of Hematology Services, Memorial Sloan-Kettering Cancer Center; Barrie Cassileth, Ph.D., chief, Integrative Medicine at Memorial Sloan-Kettering Cancer Center.

To our agent, Jonathan Dolger, whose first enthusiasm launched the plan of action, thank you for remaining calm during our many questions and concerns, and to Jane Isay for your kind words of advice. Many thanks to our editor, Marnie Cochran at Perseus, for her vision and focus.

With special appreciation to Alison Freeland, without whom this would never be. You have taken a complex subject and made it into a simple and uplifting story to tell. For your long-distance communication and patience with e-mails and Word documents without viruses, cheers.

Much appreciation to my family; my parents, Audrey and Harold, for their consistent "go-for-it" mantra, my brother Brian for his support and reinforcement, and especially to Steve, for his encouragement, laughter, and love.